# Transformation of the Heart:

*Tales of the Profound Impact Therapy Dogs Have on Their Humans*

Teri Pichot, LCSW, MAC, LAC

iUniverse, Inc.
New York   Bloomington

# Transformation of the Heart

## Tales of the Profound Impact Therapy Dogs Have on Their Humans

iUniverse books may be ordered through booksellers or by contacting:

iUniverse
1663 Liberty Drive
Bloomington, IN 47403
www.iuniverse.com
1-800-Authors (1-800-288-4677)

ISBN: 978-1-4401-2986-5 (pbk)
ISBN: 978-1-4401-2987-2 (cloth)
ISBN: 978-1-4401-2988-9 (ebk)

Printed in the United States of America

iUniverse rev. date: 03/25/2009

Also by Teri Pichot:

*Solution-Focused Substance Abuse Treatment*
(with Sara Smock)

*Animal-Assisted Brief Therapy: A Solution-Focused Approach*
(with Marc Coulter)

*Solution-Focused Brief Therapy: Its Effective Use in Agency Settings*
(with Yvonne Dolan)

*To Rockefeller and Jasper,*
*the best therapists a person could ever have.*

The stories contained in this book are from the perspectives of the therapy dog handlers who told them to me. The stories are not meant to be historically accurate; I am simply reporting them as told to me by the handlers. I conducted the majority of interviews at the sites the therapy dog team visits, and in many cases, family members or other professionals confirmed some of the facts. In addition, each handler generously reviewed my draft to ensure that I used these interviews accurately. The therapy dog handlers have disclosed significant personal information, and on occasion have requested that specific facts be modified for the purpose of protecting their privacy. I have also modified names of clients and other facts to maintain privacy.

# Contents

# Illustrations

# Foreword

A remark by Roger Caras, a past president of the American Society for the Prevention of Cruelty to Animals, "Dogs are not our whole life, but they make our lives whole," seems very apropos as an introduction to this Foreword. His use of the word wholeness is intriguing, perhaps because of its direct implication to understanding the human-animal bond. Living with animals can complete people. This loving bond between humans and animals can make wonderful contributions to our quality of life.

A growing body of research demonstrates that animals can promote human physical and emotional wellness simply by being part of our lives. The research has demonstrated the healing impact of animals on humans facing various physical and emotional challenges. These findings lend a strong impetus for establishing animal-assisted interventions.

Many say their connection with animals makes them feel fulfilled. Just watch people play, walk, or just sit next to their adored pets and you can personally witness that sense of wholeness. When I ask people about their pets, so many share their feelings, not only with words, but with a warm glow that comes from deep within their souls. It's a glow you can actually feel. Their commentaries are usually filled with stories about lives that are blessed with the pleasure, love, and affection that their pets bring to them.

Perhaps the most critical ingredient creating wholeness is the intimacy that is established in our relationships with animals. Anyone who has loved an animal knows what I mean when I say intimate. It is the spark in the eyes when you connect; it is the "vavoom" that is generated when two souls touch each other, and we are bewitched.

You are about to read a very warm-hearted book, *Transformation of the Heart,* that provides a unique glimpse into the relationships established between therapy animals and human companions on a daily basis. This book contains a collection of stories told by individuals who have learned the power of partnering with a loving canine. Each story not only tells the tale of a therapy dog's job of visiting others, but it also sheds light on the impact of the dog's life on his/her partner. The book incorporates engaging, heartwarming stories of eighteen therapy dogs and their relationships with their partners. Teri has taken great attention to provide you with a tender glimpse that helps you understand how those who volunteer with their animals are also touched by their therapy dogs. It is only natural that as family pets these animals may also provide support to their partners, just like any loving pet owner may experience.

It is common for people to volunteer in activities that mirror their interests and lifestyles. Many volunteer in areas where they find passion in their lives for personal reasons or sometimes just for altruism. Many who have a fondness for animals may find themselves volunteering in programs that serve animals, or utilize animals in positive ways, including animal-assisted interventions. Some may volunteer in a service project where they once found some hope themselves and had some personal gain. It is only logical that many who have witnessed the power of the human-animal bond in their personal lives would be excellent ambassadors to share those outcomes with others.

What you typically find in books about animal-assisted interventions (AAI) are chapters that focus on how the bond is formulated, chapters on how these interventions should be established, and chapters about the concerns and safeguards of incorporating animals into various special populations. Numerous other books on AAI act as testimonies filled with warmhearted stories that illustrate and document the miraculous victories and outcomes witnessed.

In *Transformation of the Heart*, Teri focuses on what I would call the back stories, accounts that not only tell the tales of therapy outcomes but focus on how these endearing animals impact the lives of their partners. The narratives you will read could be about any of us. They are about people who are devoted to their individual animals and are willing to share that love with many others.

The chapters are filled with remarkably moving stories. For example, you will have the chance to read about a white Labrador retriever named Avalanche and her relationship with her human partner, Susan. Although Avalanche was deeply bonded to Susan's husband, that suddenly changed after a family vacation. The story shows how Susan's relationship with Avalanche and her volunteer work helped her overcome her sense of loss and build a new life.

In an additional chapter, you will read a story of a big orange Newfoundland mix, Molly, who was rescued by a woman named Emily. The story explores the lessons that Emily learned by working with Molly. Molly showed Emily the power of small acts of kindness and inspired her to look for ways she, too, could make a small difference in the lives of others.

I waited many years to have a similar love from animals. Ironically, I grew up without family pets. Although I was curious about animals, they were not a part of my family life. In fact, I grew up being a little apprehensive about dogs. I realize now my anxieties towards them stemmed from a lack of exposure rather than any specific incidents. How lucky my life became when I found my first dog twenty-five years ago, and my life was changed forever as I learned to bond with four-legged and winged beings.

My nonhuman family members and working colleagues have had a dramatic impact on my working life. They have had a tremendous influence on supporting my young charges. These animals have been influential in opening doors that appeared shut and providing clients with a blanket of emotional security that promoted strong therapeutic relationships. I started twenty-five years ago to find a miracle to help me help children, but the miracle ended up finding me. My animals' tenacity for life is indeed their greatest attribute. They appreciate every moment they have, and it's the daily ordinary moments they seem to enjoy the most. They wait at the door every day to go to work. It is part of their daily ritual, so going is expected. What is unexpected is how they relate with such endearing kindness and devotion. My initial work with therapy animals was to have them break the ice with my clients. Their role was simple: Make everyone feel comfortable and wanted. But through my experiences with my therapy dogs, I also have learned about life. Just like in many of the stories you are about to read, my animals have brought out the best in me, and they have taught me many lessons about others and myself. The animals I share my life with have taught me to be calm, gentle, and, ironically, to act more "human and humane" with others.

I could also share back-stories about how my animals have made my life and those of other members of my family richer. I could tell you how our therapy animals mentored my boys through their childhood or how our youngest dog, Magic, was the strongest source of support to my wife when she was recovering from her breast cancer surgery. But *Transformation of the Heart* isn't about my stories, but rather the kindhearted stories of many other men and women whose narratives about their relationship with their animals you are about to read.

The belief that dogs make our lives whole is a truth that we must cherish and celebrate. We shouldn't glamorize their contributions with exaggerated praise, but let our admiration be based on honest observations which will support these beliefs. Some say that pet companions are lucky that we take care of them. We will soon learn once again how far from the truth that is. We are the lucky ones! You are about to read and hear stories that will capture your heart. I know, because I was touched as well.

Aubrey H. Fine, Ed.D.
Professor, California Poly University
Licensed Psychologist
Author, *Afternoons with Puppy* and the *Handbook on Animal Assisted Therapy*

# Acknowledgements

I would like to say a very special thank you to all of the therapy dog handlers who took the time to contact me and tell me their stories. Each is amazingly special in his or her own way, and it was an honor to meet them all. I appreciate their patience with my many questions and their willingness to share their personal lives with all of us. Without them, this book would not have been possible.

Writing a book such as this requires tremendous behind-the-scene support, and I am truly grateful for all who helped make this book possible. Yvonne Dolan called me one summer afternoon and asked if I would be willing to write a book about therapy dogs and their stories of healing. It was this phone call that started the ball rolling and instigated my exciting journey meeting therapy dogs and their handlers across the country. She has remained a tremendous supporter of my work, and an invaluable sounding board throughout this process. A special thank you to Diana McQuarrie for her help spreading the news throughout the therapy dog community about my need for stories. She has remained a quiet supporter of my work, for which I am very grateful.

On a more personal level, a heartfelt thank you to Mark Hochstedler, Ashley Foster, Calyn Crow, and Charlie Johnson. Mark is my dear husband and friend. He created and maintains my Web site, which encouraged people to contact me to share all these wonderful therapy dog stories and connects me to my readers, and he gave up countless days together to allow me the time

7

each weekend to complete this project. He became the family chef on my writing days to ensure we didn't starve, catered to the canine family members' requests, and helped around the house to keep the fur balls and dust bunnies at bay. I'm sure I don't say enough how much I appreciate his love and support!

Ashley is my trusted dog expert and advocate. She generously answers questions and provides guidance each time my pups do something I don't quite understand. She is the one who gives words of encouragement each time I question my own skills and knowledge as a therapy dog handler. I know she always has my dogs' best interest at heart, and I trust her explicitly. Calyn is a true friend who spent hours helping me to catch the countless typos that are an inevitable part of writing. And last, but definitely not least, Charlie is my dear friend and mentor. He encouraged me to pursue this project during times in which it looked as if it might not be possible, reviewing my work and giving possible leads. He is always there for professional advice and wisdom. Thank you.

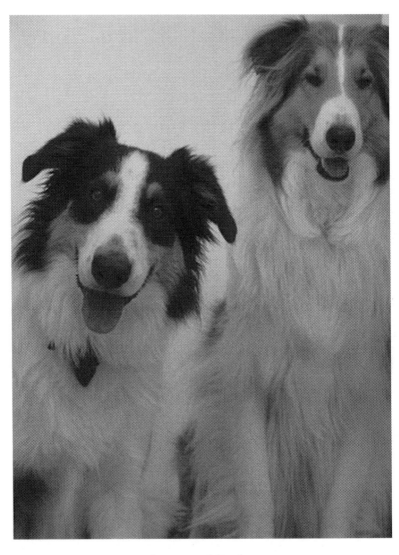

Jasper and Rocky
*Photo by Teri Pichot*

# Introduction

*Dogs mirror us back to
ourselves in unmistakable ways
that, if we are open, foster true
understanding and change.*

—The Monks of New Skete

Even when one is grown, it can be challenging to perfect the
mother-daughter relationship. Transitioning from the hierarchical
parent-child structure to something more mutually supportive
is a difficult journey, one that is often fraught with difficult
emotions and ungraceful interactions. Parents still have a way of
unintentionally bringing one back to past feelings and patterns
despite how many years go by. Unfortunately, I am no exception
to this inevitable developmental stage. Since my parents live in
another state, I don't get to see them as much as I would like,
so visits are special. Regrettably, this distance also minimizes the
opportunities we have together to resolve this life transition. Any
time my parents are able to get away to Colorado to visit, it is a
special time, and I do my best to make it memorable. I scramble
to get the housework done, plan special menus, and look forward
to having them join in our family routines.

Part of normal growing up is sifting through everything we
were taught in order to decide who we really are. This means
evaluating all of the values, choices, and ways of doing things
that we are taught in childhood. It is necessary for each of us to
determine who we are and what fits best. This setting aside of
past values and ways of doing things and developing a uniquely
new path only adds to the complexity of growing up. Inevitably,
this means that we will have many similarities to our parents,
but also many differences. Now that I am in my forties, I'm very

comfortable with my life, values, and ways of interacting in the world. I think I have done well with that part of growing up. Unfortunately, I have not yet mastered how to be completely comfortable being me around my parents; specifically around my mother's occasional comments about my choices. Now, I don't believe she is purposefully judging my choices, but she does have that motherly tone that still has a way of letting me know she would do things quite differently.

One of the ways that I chose to be different from my upbringing was in my love of and devotion to dogs. In my childhood home, a dog's place was in the backyard in a designated dog run. This prevented our dog from ruining the lawn and other landscaping, destroying our belongings, soiling the carpet, etc. When I was young, this worked out well, since I enjoyed the outdoors and was happy to join our dog in her pen to play. However, as I became older, I found it difficult to choose between time with my pet and indoor activities. I longed to include my dog in all of my activities. I vowed that this would be something I would do differently when I was an adult. True to that promise, I did. I have had a dog all of my adult life, and those dogs have always been house dogs. Muddy (and worse) tracks through the house, scratches on the wood floors, hair on my clothes and everything else, and even the occasional disgusting bodily fluid on brand new carpet have been well worth it to have my pets take a central place in our home. There is nothing better than curling up with the pups and husband to settle in for a good movie. It just wouldn't be home without them. Similar to my conclusions about my husband, my dogs are well worth the occasional mess and property loss.

So you can just imagine the cognitive dissonance when my parents come to visit. They have come to terms with the fact that the dogs will be in the house, but I can feel my mother's stress level rise as my gorgeous sable and white collie assists her in sorting through the vegetable bin in the fridge while preparing dinner or when he politely sniffs my niece's son's toys to see what he brought as entertainment. Now it is important to note that my two collies are very well trained. Both are registered therapy dogs who[1] work with me at a local substance abuse treatment center. However, they are still dogs, and are far from perfect. They are curious, playful, and very furry. In addition, collies are notorious for leaving drool spots on the floor and everywhere else. Jasper (my younger, tri-color collie mix) loves to play and continuously offers his toys in an invitation to engage in a game of tug or fetch. In order to reinforce their curiosity (a very important trait for a therapy dog), I welcome their involvement. They are welcome to sniff anything new that enters the house, and they expect to be a part of most activities. This flies in the face of my upbringing in which dogs were considered to be somewhat dirty (which made sense when they were forced to remain outside). I am a sensitive soul, and I do my best to minimize the stress my parents feel when they visit, yet I also seek to be true to who I am. Finding this optimal balance can be a tall order.

Dogs are incredible. They are experts on their humans and have a way of knowing immediately if anything is amiss. While I can normally hide my nervous anticipation from my husband and parents, my dogs automatically know something is up. This is especially true for my older dog, Rocky. Rocky and I are very much alike. We are both highly sensitive, perfectionist, prefer to have our environment remain somewhat constant, and are a little anxious around change. While I do my best to keep these emotions under wraps, Rocky barfs and gets diarrhea when stressed. So, needless to say, just when I am already stressed, Rocky has a humbling way of expressing his emotions in an unavoidable way. This brings us to my parents' visit one summer.

---

1 Although grammatically animals are referred to as "that," I have purposefully chosen to disregard this grammatical rule on many occasions throughout this book and refer to animals as "who" due to their central role in our lives and in the purpose of Animal-Assisted Activities/Therapy.

Two days before they were scheduled to arrive, Rocky suddenly began vomiting while at work. At first I didn't worry, since he has a sensitive stomach and an occasional episode is par for the course. Rocky gives plenty of warning before he vomits, and he is trained to use the trash can (with some prompting) to minimize any mess in the workplace. Rocky had a fairly low-key day, so I took him off duty and he rested in my office as I finished up my work. As the day progressed, so did his vomiting. By the end of the day I was becoming worried, so I contacted his veterinarian and scheduled an appointment for the following day. It's always hard to see my pet so sick. Rocky didn't understand why I was insisting that he eat ice cubes or why I suddenly shoved a bowl in front of his face as he began to heave in the middle of the night. Luckily, the vet's diagnosis, while not specific, was not overly worrisome. She stated that we had staved off the serious complication of dehydration, and that Rocky most likely had caught a bug or eaten something that didn't agree with him. With medicine and canned food for a bland diet in hand, I was confident we were on the mend. All would be on schedule for my family's arrival.

The following day was beautiful! A classic Colorado summer day. I hurried to get the house clean before my parents' arrival, as Jasper slunk from room to room doing his best to avoid the horrid vacuum cleaner while still remaining close to me as I cleaned. Rocky seemed irritated that I kept insisting he move as I did my best to clean around and under him as he followed me throughout the home. With the house clean at last, I took a moment to enjoy the fur-free floors, knowing that it was just a matter of minutes before tuffs of collie fur would again whimsically float across the wooden floors at the slightest breeze. Part of collie ownership is being at peace with a home that always shows some evidence that dogs are part of the family. Even so, I always find a sense of accomplishment in those brief moments before it all starts again. Within hours, the house was full of happy chatter as family arrived and the long awaited visit was under way. Jasper playfully assumed the role of host as he accompanied my dad to the guest room to help him settle in, and Rocky assisted my mom and me as we took the fresh peaches they had brought for canning to spread them out to finish ripening in the basement. It was then that I was reminded of my mom's uneasiness with a dog involved in household activities. Rocky's curiosity was apparent as we gathered the peaches from the boxes. He sniffed each peach, his tail gently wagging as he gave his relaxed doggy smile. He was clearly happy as he surveyed the situation and shared the excitement of the moment. Despite her discomfort, my mother's efforts to accept the different way of engaging in household tasks were clearly apparent as she came to realize that Rocky had no desire to eat the peaches or harm them in any way. It was simply a very different environment. Then, when all was going so well, it happened. My husband yelled, "Teri! Grab a towel, Jasper just threw up." Just when I was comfortable that my parents were starting to accept that dogs were a part of our everyday family, the gross and disgusting part of dog ownership reared its ugly head. There was no way to make this look good. Clearly we now had the correct diagnosis of Rocky's former ailment. It was a virus. A contagious virus, one that his younger brother now had and was going to spew all over in front of my parents! Great! Let the fun begin!

The following day started out well. Both dogs were on their best behavior, and all of us were enjoying catching up and spending time together. After a family outing, we returned home. As I opened the door, I quickly retreated. Jasper's vomiting the night before was evidently not a one-time occurrence. After instructing my parents to enter the house through an alternative door so that I could mop up the foul mess, I felt my anxiety rising. This was precisely why my parents did not think dogs should be in the house. What a perfect example of why my dogs were not allowed in their home for a visit. I took a deep breath and reminded myself that I am an adult. I can and do make different choices and, while having dogs in the home may result in me never having a perfectly clean house, the dogs are nevertheless worth it. Despite my futile attempts to cheer myself up, I didn't feel any better.

After lunch we decided to go for a walk in the neighborhood. I had been enjoying daily walks with the dogs during the summer, and they had been exhibiting model behavior as they enthusiastically ran from smell to smell to explore their world. I expected today to be no exception, and I looked forward to sharing a relaxing walk with my parents, husband, and dogs. However, true to how the visit had begun, we could not have been more than five minutes away from home when Rocky suddenly stopped to do his business. Then, to my horror, I realized that Rocky had a severe case of diarrhea. Now for those of you who are not familiar with rough coat collies, let me paint you the picture. Collies have a long flowing coat that culminates with short white fur from the knees down. The coat is perfectly designed to allow them to defecate without any mess. However, when a collie has diarrhea, all bets are off in terms of cleanliness. In fact, the fur "pants," as dog experts describe the long flowing hair under the tail and around the hindquarters, is a perfect place for the liquid mess to gather. Rocky, oblivious to my desire to demonstrate to my parents that one can have dogs living peacefully in the house while still having a reasonably clean home, proceeded to walk proudly right in front of my parents with his "chocolate pants" gently blowing in the breeze. I was humiliated! I quickly found tissues and did my best to clean him up, but this only seemed to smear the smelly mess further. Just when I thought my humiliation could not be any greater, Jasper joined in.

A large German shepherd that lives in our neighborhood charged the fence toward us. Jasper in turn lunged and barked frantically. My parents both startled and began to walk rapidly away from the canine ruckus. Now, this German shepherd has a reputation in the neighborhood for biting, and the owner has several signs posted stating, "Beware of Dog." On my daily walks

I do my best to avoid this dog out of fear that he might someday get loose. However, my husband believes I am overreacting, so when we walk together, we usually walk past the German shepherd's home. This was not something that I thought wise to share with my parents at this moment, nor was it the time or place to tell my husband that I was indeed correct about the dangers of the German shepherd. Consistent with how the rest of our day had progressed, I suddenly realized that the gate to this dog's yard was wide open. I hurried Rocky and my parents past the gate, as my husband wrestled to maintain control of the very loud and scary-looking Jasper. Thankfully, the German shepherd is apparently not that bright, for he never noticed that he could have easily gone through the gate and tormented us (or worse). He huffed in defeat as we rapidly gained some distance from the yard and gathered our thoughts. Unwilling to go back the way we had come for fear that the German shepherd might somehow discover the opening, I became overwhelmed. I could not possibly imagine a worse start to our visit. I was embarrassed by Jasper's behavior. My parents were both fearful of out-of-control dogs, and I would classify my own dog in that category after his outburst. The years of obedience training and perfect manners were pushed far back in their minds. There was no way to make this look good. I stared ahead in silence at Rocky's chocolate pants. Defeat was imminent. Canine quarrels over bones and vomit on the laundry room floor was nothing compared to this. I could feel my parents' disapproval as we continued our walk. I had nothing to say.

As we returned home and we ushered Rocky into the tub for a bath, I had to laugh; there really was nothing else to do at that point. This was not the only less-than-perfect visit with my parents. On their previous visit we had to rush Rocky to the animal hospital for pneumonia on Christmas day. I cared for him on the family room floor as the rest of the family watched television. My husband and I stayed up with him all night as he vomited and had a high fever. Not the ideal Christmas.

Now, in August, as my husband and I gave Rocky a bath to clean his pants and I laughed about how life with dogs is far from predictable or glamorous, something changed deep inside of me. I found a sense of peace—if only for a moment. It was then that I realized that Rocky and Jasper's role was to help me learn to be myself, no matter how humbling or embarrassing it may be. Being comfortable being myself around those who are different from me has always been a difficult thing. As a child I quickly learned how cruel children could be, and as a result I sought to blend in to avoid the hurtful words. I carried this coping skill well into adulthood to deal with immature and thoughtless co-workers. Ironically, it was my therapy dogs' ability to assist me in being more human in social settings that I valued most. I could not help but smile more, be more playful, and ultimately to be more myself when I worked with my dogs during client sessions or visitations. However, this same trait resulted in me having to show this human side in settings for which I was not prepared. This was a difficult life lesson for me, and Rocky and Jasper could not have been better teachers. I wasn't going to live life without them, and they surely were not going to care about perceptions, gain more social skills, or any of the other unrealistic behaviors I had been secretly hoping from my dogs. They were offering me a gift that I could choose to accept. By just being themselves, they were offering me the chance to be a better human.

Rocky and Jasper are well known for their volunteer work as therapy dogs, and I receive many kind words of appreciation for the work they do to help others. Everyone assumes that their work is to help other people, and, outwardly, these assumptions are correct. However, the true day-to-day work that the boys do is to help heal me from the bumps and bruises of life. They give me enormous joy while also occasionally bringing up feelings of embarrassment and frustration to help me learn to better master these emotions. I am truly appreciative of them.

And so came the inspiration for this book. A dog's presence offers humans one of two choices: to escape from people and problems into a canine world, or to learn from our canine friends and thereby become a better human and take a more active and purposeful role in life with people. This book contains a collection of stories that have been told to me by individuals who have learned the power of partnering with a loving canine. Each story not only tells the tale of a therapy dog's job of visiting others, but it sheds light on the unique gifts each dog gives to his or her human companion every day. There is an undeniable bond between animals and humans. We need each other. While the gifts that humans give to dogs are more readily labeled (i.e., food, shelter, protection), it is time that we begin to recognize the countless gifts our working canine buddies give to us. So, settle in and invite your own family pet to snuggle next to you as you enjoy a journey into the wonderful world of therapy dogs to see how they transform the hearts of the humans they love.

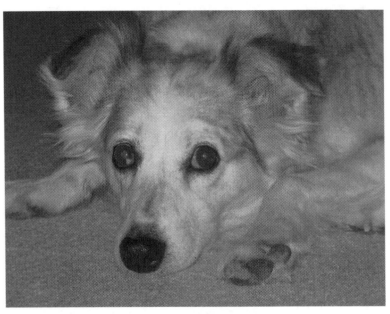

Splash
*Photo by Michelle Penfold*

# Chapter One
# Splash

*Dogs are not our whole life, but*
*they make our lives whole.*

—Roger Caras

The date was September 13, 2003. As I walked into the large open room, I felt the nervousness that was typical whenever I gathered with a group of strangers. While I had been looking forward to taking this class, I still had butterflies and was apprehensive about the unknown. I had worked hard to get to this point, and an important personal dream depended on my successful completion of this milestone. A large stuffed dog sat in the middle of the room, with a plastic bin filled with dog paraphernalia placed near by. A PowerPoint presentation was on continual play at the front of the room, showing pictures of smiling people with perfect looking canines. Stacks of books pertaining to dog training sat on the table near the plastic bin. Walkers with tennis balls adorning their feet, a wheelchair, and other equipment to help the differently-abled leaned against the front wall. At the front of the room was a friendly-looking woman glancing at her notes, and by her side lay a small, older golden retriever wearing a therapy dog vest. Wow! I thought. That will be a tough standard to meet. My dog would never be so perfect and focused with a group of strangers. He would have immediately wanted to run say hello, or, with my luck, barked to question why these people were joining us in the room. He would have then run to the walker and tried to grab it by the tennis ball in an effort to play, completely unaware that a frail person might depend on that piece of equipment for balance. This was yet another thing I had not thought to prepare my canine partner to master.

I visually scanned the room, looking for the perfect seat. Somewhere with a good view of the front of the room, but not so close that the instructor would single me out or use me for demonstrations. I learn best through observation. Unfortunately for me, many teachers do their best to mix it up, adding multiple kinds of teaching methods in an effort to reach all students. While it is good in theory (I even use that same approach when I teach), I hate interactive exercises during workshops, and I naturally look for ways to avoid them by just blending in. The tables were arranged in a horseshoe configuration, which didn't bode well for remaining a wallflower. Eager to settle in for a day-long workshop, I saw the perfect seat across the room. It was far enough away that I hoped I could avoid whatever the instructor had in store for the blindfold sitting by the stack of books. A woman close to my own age was sitting alone, looking down at the handouts. She had an inviting warmth about her, so I grabbed a water bottle and a package of handouts and made my way across the room. After polite introductions, I settled into my seat. Her name was Michelle, and she quickly told me all about her five-year-old Aussie/border collie mix, Splash. I smiled as she quickly brought out pictures of her pride and joy and rattled on about what a great therapy dog she thought she would be. She was incredibly easy to talk to; just what I needed to help me relax and be more comfortable. Before long she had me showing pictures of my own dog, and we became lost in swapping stories about our pups, our hopes, and our dreams.

Before long it was time for the class to begin, and despite my efforts to blend in, I soon learned that was not going to be possible sitting next to my new friend. Michelle's easygoing nature also meant that she was quick to volunteer answers or to be a part of exercises. She seemed completely comfortable within her own skin, and she quickly engaged in conversations and volunteered during breaks to help improve the instructor's handouts and PowerPoint presentations for future workshops. She did it all in such a non-intrusive manner that she somehow became an integral part of this new organization before even passing the upcoming exam. It was a gift that I truly envied and I wondered how some people seemed to escape the dreaded curse of social anxiety that I faced.

During lunch, Michelle and I discussed our dogs and confided our fears that our beloved pets might not measure up to the strict Delta Society standards despite our best efforts to train and prepare. Although I hoped for the best for Michelle in the upcoming exam, I was secretly relieved to hear that I was not alone in thinking my pet might have difficulty tolerating some of the crowding or noisy situations that were simulated in the exam. The therapy dogs in the video tapes, and the already registered therapy dogs who came into the classroom to demonstrate the visit scenarios, seemed so perfectly trained; their normal canine nature mysteriously absent or controlled. None demonstrated the short attention span and cautiousness that I saw in Rocky. I strongly believed my dog could be great as a therapy dog, but I could not picture him instinctively knowing how to handle new and challenging situations, or approaching odd looking equipment to initiate a visit with an infirm person like the dogs before me did. Rocky seemed to carry his flaws on his shoulder, with no ability to hide his true being. This being said, I was both surprised and relieved when Michelle told me that Splash was a submissive pee-er. Finally, a dog with a flaw! It somehow gave me hope that just maybe some flaws would be acceptable in this new world of working canines.

The workshop was soon over, and our examination times were set for two weeks later. The workshop gave us both the hope and energy we needed to take the next steps, and Michelle had even decided to have her horse, Spyderman, take the exam as well. Michelle and I parted ways, but not before exchanging e-mail addresses and wishing each other well. Our exams were scheduled back to back, so I knew our paths would cross again.

The next two weeks were a blur of training, grooming, and nervousness as the therapy dog exam approached. Before long, test day arrived. Rocky, Splash, and even Spyderman all somehow passed, much to our relief. We were officially Delta Society Pet Partners. Michelle's and my paths crossed on occasion after that. There were the occasional e-mails, or monthly therapy dog meetings, and a Christmas party. I became lost in my own work with my canine friend, and Michelle moved on with her own life. Each time I spoke with Michelle, I was struck by how confident she was in her work with Splash. I even once saw Michelle in a wheelchair at a therapy dog meeting following knee surgery, with Splash dutifully by her side. They truly looked the part of a seasoned, confident, perfectly trained therapy dog-handler team. Splash had blossomed. Each time I saw Michelle, she was right in the middle of the activities of the therapy dog organization. She seemed so confident and in her element.

As the years went by, I lost contact with Michelle. She was no longer with the local therapy dog association chapter, and I no longer had time to attend the functions that had caused our paths to cross. Imagine my surprise when one evening on the 10:00 p.m. news, there were Michelle and Splash, featured in a story about service dogs. A service dog? How could that be? "Rocky!" I said to my sleeping collie. "There's your buddy Splash!" He dutifully lifted his head in the direction of the television, turned to look at me in confusion, and then resumed his nap, as I watched intently. I wondered if the headline was just another example of the media misunderstanding the difference between a therapy dog and a service dog. But then I learned that my friend suffers from *trichotillomania*, an impulse-control disorder in which the person frequently pulls out one's own hair to cope with anxiety, leading to noticeable hair loss. How could I have not even noticed that! Michelle never exhibited any signs of anxiety; in fact she was the exact opposite in her confident demeanor. I quickly found her e-mail address and asked if I could come interview her for a book I was writing about the surprising ways in which therapy dogs help their own handlers. She obliged and an appointment was set.

It was a cold winter day as I parked my car outside of the medical center where Michelle and Splash now work. Yet as they came around the corner to greet me, it was like the day I first met Michelle. She exuded warmth and confidence, and I instantly felt comfortable. Splash ran up and quickly rolled over so I could scratch her belly as her tail wagged and she gave me her characteristic doggy smile. Soon we were in Michelle's office, and Splash leaned against my leg and occasionally nudged my hand to remind me to pet her as Michelle told her story.

It all began when Michelle was three years old, and she was attacked by the family's Saint Bernard. Soon after, she started pulling her doll's hair out, and then progressed to her own, pulling it out strand by strand. As we talked, Michelle lifted her hair up to show me patches of new hair growth and explained that the hair grows back more curly than the original; resulting in patches that she refers to as "carpet." It was a secret that resulted in her feeling alone, like no one could possibly understand. Anxiety became part of her everyday life. She tried everything, and nothing worked. Finally, she realized the goal was simply to manage the symptoms; there was no cure.

In 2004 she accepted a position as the volunteer services manager for the medical center. It was a dream job, and got her back doing the work she had done twenty years before. She was able to bring Splash with her to work, and she worked with other therapy dog teams to help change the lives of patients and staff. Her professional life was falling into place, and she could not have been happier. Then the unexpected happened.

One day when she was talking to Pat, one of the volunteers who happened to train services dogs, Pat said, "Do you see what Splash is doing?" Only then did Michelle began to realize that, at the very moment Michelle began to experience anxiety and pull her hair, Splash moved in to nudge her right hand so Michelle would pet her instead. It was then that Michelle realized she only pulled her hair with her right hand, never her left. At these precise moments of anxiety, Splash would nudge her right hand—again, never her left. Splash somehow knew how to provide the distraction Michelle needed to make her hair pulling a conscious behavior, thereby making it something that Michelle could control. It was an intervention I knew well as a psychotherapist and frequently encouraged in my clients. It's called "pattern interruption." Often people do things out of habit, and therefore have little chance to change the unconscious behavior, for it occurs before the person has a chance to respond. If the person can simply find something to interrupt the habit or pattern, the person now has the option of choosing to do something different, thereby forming a new habit. It's a simple concept, and one that Splash had seemed to master unbeknownst to her human partner. It was ingenious, and something that no professional could have possibly devised. Yet it was so natural and instinctual to Splash.

Michelle went on to tell me that Splash also had found a way to remind Michelle to take her medication. Each morning when Michelle reaches for her toothbrush, Splash quickly appears and begins to nudge Michelle. Splash's simple presence reminds her it is time to take her medication.

And so Michelle began the process of working with Splash to become a certified service dog, so that Splash could legally accompany her everywhere to do these jobs the dog had created. With the newfound confidence Splash had found through her work as a therapy dog, she was able to pass her service dog test with ease. Splash takes her job very seriously and has now traveled on airplanes, trains, etc., with Michelle and has had many adventures as a service dog.

Splash also has ways of finding who she is meant to help. Michelle told me about a woman whom she and Splash once visited at the medical center. The team was walking through the hospital when Splash suddenly began to pull toward a woman sitting alone. Michelle followed Splash toward the woman, and soon Splash was nudging the woman's hand to say hello. As the woman looked to Michelle as though to question Splash's presence, Michelle simply said, "Splash found you." Splash then put her front paws up on the client (something that Splash rarely does), and the woman embraced the dog and began to weep. Michelle later learned that this woman was going to surgery and was extremely stressed. We may never know the difference that visit from Splash made for the woman that day, but Splash knew this was a woman she could help.

As my chat with Michelle drew to a close, I couldn't help but glance at the photographs on her bookshelf. There was Spyderman, proudly wearing his Delta Society vest. (I must admit I had never seen a horse in a therapy horse vest before.) Next to Spyderman's photo was a picture of Splash in her service dog vest, beside a face I didn't recognize. "That's Rusty," Michelle said, referring to the red heeler in the picture. "He's new. He just showed up one day, and I found myself asking, 'Could he be my next therapy dog?'" Michelle went on to explain that she believes that all of her animals come to her for a reason. She has discovered Splash's reason, and now she is working to train Rusty to be both a therapy and service dog. His reason will someday become clear.

Michelle has learned so much from Splash. "She is a great teacher," she explained. Splash is the reason Michelle renewed her connection to her community and returned to her work as a volunteer manager. She has even worked with others in the area to found a group of Delta Society Pet Partners called the Colorado Therapy Animals. Together, Splash and Michelle are now touching the lives of others.

Splash is no longer a submissive pee-er now that she has found her role in life. Michelle went on to explain how, by working together, Splash now understands that Michelle will protect her no matter what. There's no reason to fear. As I listened, I found myself silently hoping that Rocky felt the same about working with me. Both Splash and Michelle are now more confident, each able to conquer their inner demons with the help of the other. They are both better off as a result of their relationship.

Michelle and Splash are a perfect example of the secret truth that lies within each therapy dog's heart. While Michelle and Splash visit clients as part of their daily job and outwardly work miracles, there is a secret that those whom they visit will never know. Those around them believe that Michelle and Splash are solely there to make their day a little better through a therapy dog visit, when in reality Michelle and Splash heal each other in the process.

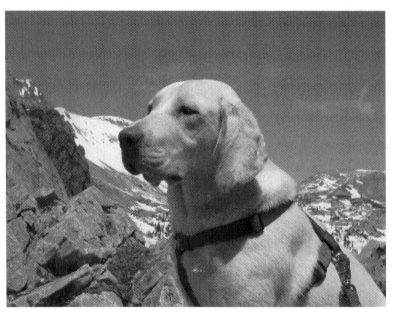

Avalanche
*Photo by Susan Deniston*

# Chapter Two
# Avalanche

*It's no coincidence that man's
best friend cannot talk*

—Anonymous

Friends. They play such a pivotal role in our lives. They are not family, yet for many, friends find a way into that cherished inner circle. Most of us met our best friends by happenstance, never knowing when we first met how close we would become nor for how long. Friends are like valuable gems upon which we stumble during our journey called life. Each friendship is wonderfully unique. Some people have been best friends from childhood while others have been best friends for only a few short months or years. Watching best friends interact, one can never tell the length of the relationship nor its future course. It is as if some friends' paths were destined to cross. For some, these relationships endure for a lifetime, yet for others, their paths part ways again, leaving each irrevocably changed for the better. It is when these friendships split apart that one can truly appreciate the resiliency inherent in all of life. Despite the loss of a cherished friendship, new friends are found and new relationships forged. However, new friends never replace old. Each friend is unique and each holds a special place in one's heart. This is the story of Avalanche.

Avalanche was one of a litter of seven tiny Labrador retriever pups. Susan's husband, Joe, had the idea to breed their chocolate lab, August, but it was only by happenstance that she met the perfect dog to stud Auggie. She was taking a leisurely walk one day when she noticed a beautiful chocolate lab swimming as his owner proudly watched from the shoreline. Instantly, she realized that the dog was Auggie's perfect match, and she quickly

31

approached the gentleman about the possibility of breeding their two labs. The owner confided that he also had been considering the possibility of breeding his dog, and he readily agreed to the plan once he learned that Auggie was already in heat. Approximately sixty-three days later, Auggie showed signs of labor. Susan carefully prepared a quiet, secluded location, and at 1:00 a.m. one September morning with Susan and her seventeen-year-old son watching in awe, Auggie whelped seven gorgeous puppies—five chocolate, one yellow, and one pure white. Although the agreement was that the owner of the stud dog would have first pick of the litter, he declined, saying that he would wait until their second litter. Unfortunately that day never came, since Auggie miscarried during their next attempt years later, and Susan called it quits in order to protect Auggie's health.

Ironically, it was Joe who had made it clear prior to breeding Auggie that they were not to keep any of the puppies. They simply did not need another dog. However, despite his strong utterances, the uniqueness of the pure white pup was too hard to resist. It was Joe, supported by his children, who led the pleas to keep the tiny pup, and Susan soon succumbed to their persistence. Soon Joe and the white pup he named Avalanche were inseparable. He chose the name Avalanche due to the rushing sound she made as she raced down the stairs in a blur of white. Each night Avalanche would bark until Joe finally gave in and let her lay on top of him in his favorite chair. There they snuggled as they enjoyed an evening of togetherness and whatever was on the television that night. Avalanche soon became a fixture of their window and door store as she accompanied Joe to work each morning. She lay underneath his big oak desk in the showroom, and Joe even cut a hole in the desk to ensure Avalanche could survey the showroom from her vantage point. They enjoyed regular hiking and fishing trips. Even though Avalanche was less than impressed with the boat rides, she was loyal to a fault and she dutifully stayed by her friend's side. Susan and Joe never put much thought into formal obedience training. There was no need. Avalanche and the labs who preceded her received on the job training in the door and window shop, and the regular stream of customers provided ample socialization. There was rarely a need for a leash, since the family business was adjacent to their residence. Avalanche learned to stay when told, and readily learned appropriate etiquette around humans. She was the model dog.

A little over a year later, Joe and Susan were looking forward to a well-deserved vacation. It was a much-anticipated annual event. As a reward for selling their quota, they packed their bags to meet up with their window supplier and other window resellers for six days in Los Cabos, Mexico. Their son had just turned eighteen, and so they decided to bring him along to celebrate this milestone while their daughter stayed behind to attend her high school classes. Leaving the frigid temperatures and snow of winter for the warm sunny beaches of Cabo San Lucas Bay was a welcome treat. As they landed after a flight of more than three hours, they were struck by the beauty of the Sea of Cortez. The native cacti and palm trees were framed on one side by the untamed waters and on the other by Cabo San Lucas's trademark rock arch. It was a stunning testament to desert beauty.

Cabo San Lucas proved to be the ideal vacation spot, as they enjoyed water sports, beaches, shopping, and socializing with friends and colleagues. Joe and their son loved Jet Skiing, one of their favorite activities, racing along the white tops of the ocean waves at top speed; enjoying the freedom and natural high it provided. While Susan accompanied them and a friend on their first trip, she preferred the more laid-back environment of the warm, relaxing beaches. So it was no surprise when on the last day of their vacation she encouraged them to go Jet Skiing without her as she enjoyed an engaging book at the water's edge.

Then the unexpected happened, something that one never thinks could ever occur when vacationing, and a risk that is never mentioned on the tranquil vacation brochures. Susan had been enjoying her book for about an hour, when suddenly a stranger came running up to her, clearly distraught as he frantically explained that there had been a tragic accident on the water. Two Jet Skis had collided at high speed, leaving her husband horribly injured. Other helpful strangers were rushing him to a local hospital, and the man said he would take Susan to meet Joe and her son. Shaken, she gathered her things and hurried after the kind stranger. Thoughts raced through her mind in nonsensical order. Dread and fear intermingled as she blindly put one foot in front of the other.

One rarely thinks much about the available medical care in foreign countries; however, this concern now became a reality for Susan. Many of the hospitals in Cabo San Lucas are much older and smaller than their equivalents in the United States, and the equipment is frequently less advanced. Spanish is the predominate language of the region, increasing the potential chaos that is likely to occur for an English speaker when tragedy strikes. Luckily, Susan's family was taken to the hospital that was best equipped to manage trauma, and the majority of the medical staff was bilingual, eliminating the language barrier. Susan's son, soaked through from the ocean and disheveled from the rescue efforts, rushed to her when their eyes met in the hospital corridor. Relieved to see her son safe, the two embraced as tears flowed freely. Then her greatest fears were confirmed. Her beloved Joe, her life partner for thirty years, could not be saved. Six hours after arriving at the hospital, he died with her at his side.

There, far away from home and stricken with grief, Susan began to sort through the myriad details required to begin the journey home to bury her husband. Despite adamant witness accounts that the death was the result of a tragic accident, well intentioned Mexican police officers struggled to determine if criminal charges should be filed against the American vacationer who accidentally hit Joe as Joe unwittingly turned sharply in front of his Jet Ski. The threat of international legal questions and red tape only added to Susan's fears as she struggled to accept the loss of her husband and to comfort her son. Through it all, kindhearted medical staff did their best to console Susan and her son, protecting the American target and thereby thwarting further legal investigation.

Through it all, a dear friend and colleague remained in Mexico with Susan and her son, securing a connection with the American Embassy and finding a local lawyer to ensure their safe exit with Joe's ashes, and helping to secure full payment for the damaged Jet Ski and the hospital bill. In addition, one unexpected person also stood by her side. That person was Oscar, the owner of the Jet Skis. Touched by the tragedy, he became their ally as he navigated the Mexican system and fought on their behalf. Susan and her son spent those days walking the beaches and contemplating their sudden loss. In retrospect, Susan now believes this was the beginning of her healing.

Back home, Susan's sixteen-year-old daughter, Ashley, bravely took on the task of planning her father's funeral in preparation for her family's return. It was a task for which no teenager could ever be prepared, but she did her father proud; she even sang the song "I Hope you Dance" through her tears at the funeral.

For Susan and her children, life had to go on. She found needed structure by running the family business on her own, and Ashley's school activities kept her involved in the world. These activities prevented Susan from staying in bed and drowning in her sorrow. She stayed strong in public, but in private, it was Avalanche who truly understood the depth of her pain. She, too, had lost her best friend. Avalanche's family had returned from the much-anticipated vacation brokenhearted and without her best friend, Joe. With Avalanche Susan could cry without any offered words of comfort. She could bury her face in Avalanche's soft white fur in silence, and they could mourn together. Avalanche soon understood she had a new best friend in Susan.

Susan found comfort in Avalanche's presence, and they

became inseparable. Living in a small town afforded Susan the opportunity of bringing Avalanche into the local bank and other businesses. Having Avalanche by her side provided the comfort and security she needed as she continued her life. Bank tellers and other professionals began to stock dog treats in anticipation of Avalanche's visits, even playfully chastising Susan when she came alone. Each summer, Susan and Joe had always had a booth at the county fair to advertise their business, and Avalanche and Susan attended the fair that summer as they had in the past. Each year Avalanche sat in her black chair as a line of visitors formed to pet her. Avalanche was well known in the community, and brought customers to the booth as children and adults alike waited patiently to visit with the dog. As Susan chatted with the booth visitors, a woman from a local hospital inquired why Susan and Avalanche were not visiting patients at the hospital, given Avalanche's popularity. Susan had never heard of therapy dogs before, and that conversation piqued her interest. Later that week, she pulled up the Delta Society's Web page, as the hospital volunteer had suggested, and learned more about the program. She didn't do anything more that year, but when the hospital volunteer gently prodded her about it the following year, she signed up for the two-day course to learn more.

Initially, Susan was intimidated by the seemingly flawless dogs used for demonstrations during the workshops. How could Avalanche ever compare? She had never taken any obedience classes, and those dogs seemed so perfect! Despite her fears, she completed the handlers' workshop. To review the basic commands, she worked tirelessly with Avalanche at the local pet store and practiced each night at home. With time, Avalanche mastered the lessons and was ready to take the therapy dog exam. Susan realized that the examiner wanted them to succeed when he gently suggested asking Avalanche to sit during the "neutral dog" part of the exam in order to better the odds of success.

Susan and Avalanche passed, and soon began to volunteer at the recently constructed hospital in her local town.

It was then that Susan realized that volunteering with Avalanche was just the medicine she needed to heal her own heart, for it gave her purpose outside of her work. When she was sad or overcome with grief, she would grab Avalanche's vest and they would volunteer together. "I would live here if I could," Susan confessed to me as we sat in the hospital lobby with Avalanche. Avalanche was indeed hard to resist. At seventy-four pounds, she was large enough to wrap one's arms around, and she reached up with her pinky-tan nose to give me kisses on my cheek as she sat sidesaddle on her right hip. Throughout our time together, visitors approached Susan and Avalanche. Many times, Susan commented, "That's one of my customers," as the person walked away. It soon became apparent that Susan's work and volunteer life intersected at the hospital as it oftentimes does in smaller towns. One visitor told Susan proudly they were visiting their new grandson that morning. Others took a moment to visit with Avalanche and give Susan a hug after a few moments of greeting.

A nurse stopped by to visit with Avalanche and Susan on her way to grab some lunch at the cafeteria. She spontaneously started talking to Susan about the wolf spider her children had recently "adopted," describing how she had gone to the local pet store to try to find appropriate nourishment. She then quickly turned to me to explain that her children adopt any animal that comes their way. Her own dog had died a short time ago, and she said that visiting with Avalanche was a part of her day that she truly enjoyed. As she left, she asked Susan what kind of dog treats she could bring for Avalanche for their next visit. No sooner had the nurse moved on than a visually impaired pregnant woman and her partner came into the waiting room. Her pink robe and endearing Christmas slippers sporting playful holiday-clad penguins spoke to her role as a current patient. Her partner lovingly guided her to a nearby chair as he quietly described Avalanche to her. Her face suddenly lit up as she turned toward us and told us about her sixty-pound lab and how strange it was not to have her canine partner with her. She proudly told us she was expecting a baby girl and that she had brought her seeing-eye dog with her to her Lamaze classes, but the nurses had asked her to leave her dog at home for the actual delivery. She seemed to enjoy Avalanche's presence all the more in the absence of her own canine friend. She and her partner then turned to enjoy the Jell-o snack they had just purchased from the cafeteria, and Susan and I continued our chat.

No sooner had we resumed our conversation than a young boy walked behind our chairs with his father, carrying lunch as they headed toward the elevators. As he walked, the boy's eyes never left Avalanche. The man turned to see what had caught his son's eye, then smiled and excitedly asked, "My wife is waiting for a dog to visit! Are you coming by soon?" Susan quickly turned, wrote down the patient's room number, and assured the gentleman that they would come by. As they left, Susan explained that it is a regular occurrence to receive requests for visits on their way out of the hospital. "It's hard to leave sometimes. I don't want to leave if someone wants a visit," she said. But I could tell by the tone of her voice that she thoroughly enjoys the visits as well and secretly hopes they never end.

She told me about several memorable visits with patients throughout the months. She smiled as she told me about a bag of homemade dog cookies that one of the emergency room physicians gave her one day from his daughter. On the brown bag the child had simply written, "Dear Avalanche. My dad says you help people. Love, Rachel." Susan spoke about special visits, arranged by the physicians, to patients in the Intensive Care Unit. Because of the ventilators and other apparatus, patients can rarely speak during visits. On one such visit, a tear quietly rolled down the side of the woman's face and Susan said, "She smiled with her eyes." Susan said it is fairly common for the nurses and other medical staff to simply drop to the floor with open arms as they pause for a quick snuggle with Avalanche in the hospital corridors. During such descriptions I could feel the depth of Susan's passion for this work, which was so obviously equally healing for her as for her patients.

As our conversation neared its end, my questions again turned toward Susan's personal life as I asked about her children. She laughed as she told me that her son thinks Avalanche is spoiled and that he is a little jealous of her. She then smiled as she stated that her children joke that Avalanche's picture is bigger than theirs on the family's picture wall. Her voice then became more serious as she told me that she knows her children are grateful for Avalanche, for they know their mother is fine now that she has Avalanche. Avalanche's presence has given them the freedom to move on with their lives and not worry about their mother. Susan's son still lives nearby, and he speaks with his mother often. Ashley has moved out of state to pursue her professional dreams.

A year after Joe's tragic death, Susan and her son traveled back to Cabo San Lucas. This time, it was for a journey of healing. Their friend Oscar met them at the airport and took them to their hotel. Oscar, also deeply touched by the accident, had worked hard for reimbursement from his insurance company for the Jet Ski, so that he could reimburse Susan the money she had paid for the damaged water craft. Together they traveled to all the places that previously had only held painful memories— everywhere except the beach. The pain there was just too great. They then visited the hospital and gave the staff members thank-you cards in appreciation for the care they had given to Joe. It was their way of closing that painful chapter.

Susan's family and friends played an invaluable role in helping her heal these last three years. She could not have done it without them. Yet when she spoke of the love of her canine friend, her voice softened and the difference was clear. "I got love and support from family and friends," she told me, "but I also got advice." Dogs, on the other hand, give unconditional love, "No buts or what ifs." That quiet support and friendship helped heal Susan's heart from the loss of the love of her life. And somewhere along the line, Avalanche's heart healed as well as she found a new best friend in Susan.

# Chapter Three
# Maggie

*Dogs are our link to paradise.*
*They don't know evil or*
*jealousy or discontent.*

—Milan Kundera

As a psychotherapist, I have heard many stories of sexual and physical abuse. It is relatively commonplace for clients who seek services in an effort to resolve problems in their day-to-day lives to also disclose distant childhood memories that are riddled with pain and mistreatment. These horrific pasts are frequently the breeding ground for dysfunctional adult relationships, domestic violence, addiction, depression, and poor coping skills in adult life. We know that children who have been abused experience significantly increased rates of alcoholism, drug abuse, sexual promiscuity, poor boundaries, increased prevalence of mental health disorders, poor self-esteem, difficulty with trust, etc., when they enter their adolescence and adult years (Brown & Finkelhor, 1986; Kendler et. al, 2000). The more prolific and chronic the abuse, the more profound and lasting are the consequences on the human psyche.

When I was working toward my undergraduate and graduate degrees, we studied some of the most well known and disturbing cases, such as that of Sybil Isabel Dorsett (Schreiber, 1989), whose childhood of abuse resulted in the fragmentation of her personality. In the early years of my career, I worked in residential treatment settings where I was exposed to some of the more disturbed clients; the majority had histories of abuse. These clients frequently had fairly poor prognoses and a normal, fully functioning life was viewed as improbable. I later accepted a job as the clinical supervisor of an outpatient substance abuse treatment center. The majority of our clients come to us from local departments of social services, which means we face a great deal of stories of heartbreaking abuse and neglect. In all of these cases, someone learned of the abuse and the professionals intervened on the children's behalf. Services are provided to both the victims and the perpetrators as society takes a protective role.

As a professional therapist, I have learned that, by definition, my exposure is limited to those who have been determined by someone (by themselves or society) to be in need of treatment or intervention. I spent my education studying problems in order to learn how to best find solutions. People who do not need services never come to my office. This can leave professionals such as me with a jaded view at times, mistakenly believing that everyone who has been sexually or physically abused has experienced lasting consequences and is therefore in need of professional help or that everyone who has used substances problematically is in need of professional intervention in order to change this behavior.

Thankfully, researchers have challenged this notion and have discovered that a surprisingly high number of people who have experienced trauma or who have engaged in problematic behavior have the ability to recover without professional help (Cloud & Granfield, 2001). In our field, this is termed resilience or spontaneous remission (Luther & Cicchetti, 2000; Luther, Cicchetti, & Becker, 2000). Some people appear to have the ability to cope with stress and catastrophe with minimal long-term damage. Trauma and stress that result in irreparable damage for some, simply become part of other people's stories, with no apparent footprint on their current lives. This discovery that the link between painful events and long-term problems is not set in stone has had a profound impact on my professional life, causing me to embrace a way of working with clients that honors this lack of linear causality (de Shazer 1985; de Shazer 1988). And maybe it was for this very reason that I was so taken with the story of Maggie.

I have received countless e-mails over this past year in response to my request for therapy dog stories. Unfortunately, in the majority of them the handler simply wanted to tell me about how wonderful his or her therapy dog is. While I'm sure these would be interesting stories, they did not fit the theme for this book, so it has been challenging to sort through the e-mails to find the stories about how handlers have been indelibly changed because of their dogs. That is simply not the story most handlers are compelled to tell, even if they are aware of it. Then I received an e-mail from Carry, and I knew I had found something special. Her e-mail began rather cryptically, not revealing her name, and stating that she would only tell me her story if I assured her the strictest anonymity.[2] After several e-mails back and forth, she agreed to meet.

When I first met Carry, a woman in her late fifties, I was struck by how warm and friendly she was. She had a wonderfully inviting smile. It was a chilly early March day, which necessitated that we meet indoors. Unfortunately, her one hundred twenty pound Saint Bernard, Maggie, was not able to come into the building, so this was one of the few interviews during which the therapy dog did not participate.

Carry was born and raised in a tiny town in Oklahoma. She was the oldest of five siblings, and had moved to Wyoming a little over four years before our meeting. She describes herself as the "responsible one"—the one who "shouldered all the blame." As far back as she can remember she was the victim of her father's sexual advances and physical rages. In order to protect her younger sisters, she did her best to be the one he came to when abuse was imminent, for if he came to her, he would often leave

2 All names, dog breed, and identifying information have been changed to protect this wonderful woman's identity. However, the basic facts of this story remain accurate.

her little sisters alone. She confided that this sexual abuse continued throughout high school.

Her father had a way of striking terror in the children's hearts as he brutally cut the heads off their pet cats in front of them, threatening, "That's what I'm going to do to you!" Threats of violence ending with death were commonplace. On one occasion, Carry, terrified, was drawn out of the house by shouts and screams only to discover her father chasing her sister with a pitchfork through the yard. The drama ended as Carry was stabbed in the foot with the pitchfork as she ran screaming between her father and little sister to stop the mayhem. She wasn't brave, she told me. She just knew she had to protect her sister. She was the only one who would. It was this sense of obligation to protect that drew Carry to the center of violence time and time again.

On an earlier occasion Carry had watched in horror as her father put each of her crying baby sisters into burlap bags and threw them into the nearby horse water trough, threatening to drown the screaming children. As Carry ran to pull the water-soaked bags from the trough, she turned to see her mother standing dumbfounded, witness to the atrocity. Despite her mother's presence, it was Carry who dragged her baby sisters to safety and assured that they were breathing. Her father left the scene ranting in a stream of obscenities, and her mother silently disappeared from the scene as if it never occurred. On another day, Carry and two of her sisters heard screams coming from the barn only to discover that her father had cornered their youngest sister. When they ran into the barn, her father made his intentions to kill the youngest girl clear, but his plan was thwarted as Carry and her sisters formed a circle around the youngest to protect her. In a rage, her father beat the three older children until they were battered and bloody. Despite the brutal outcome, they remained proud since they had protected their little sister. On other occasions, Carry hid her siblings in the attic to protect them from her father's rages, begging them to remain quiet lest they be found and suffer the consequences.

One day she asked her mother why they stayed despite her father's tyranny. Her mother simply turned, looked Carry in the eyes, and said, "I would leave if I didn't have so many kids! What do you expect me to do?" Throughout it all, Carry held onto hope that someone would find out. She was happy when her father took her to church one day, thinking that surely someone would notice the bruises and help her, only to be horrified to find that her father planned to take her to the back room and allow some of the men from church to sexually abuse her as well. Despite the bruises and marks on her and her siblings, no one helped. "People had to have known," Carry told me. But the family moved unobstructed from small town to small town. Carry now believes her father moved the family out of fear of detection. One day at a family function her uncle confided to her, "I wish I could take you children away, but I'm afraid of your father." If a grown man was too afraid to protect them, how could a young girl hope for intervention? It was then that she lost hope that anyone would ever help. She often thought it would be better if she was dead, but she realized that would leave no one to protect her sisters.

As a child, Carry learned to depend on herself. There was no one else—not her family, not God, not anyone. She became the protector, with the goal only of survival. Late at night, she would whisper to her siblings, "Fairytales don't teach children that dragons exist. They teach children that dragons were meant to be slain." Someday their dragon would be slain, and they would survive. Someday … their pain would end.

Unfortunately, this is not a story in which a rescuer ever came. Child Protection never intervened to protect these five children. They simply grew up. The abuse stopped for her two younger sisters when they were approximately ten years old, although her father continued to abuse Carry throughout high school. She moved out of the house as soon as she graduated, but stayed close by to protect her sisters if need be. Her father had rarely harmed her two youngest siblings, a boy and a girl. Carry's father had always insisted upon having a son and stubbornly persisted in having more children until his wife conceived a boy. Ironically, he then ignored and neglected this son. The youngest girl was also more neglected than abused.

Carry's father had numerous affairs, and her mother stayed through it all. With time, Carry came to a place in which she didn't hate him, but there was no love. She realized that the father, who had once instilled fear in her heart, was no longer a threat. His spirit was broken. She was no longer afraid of him, and with time she found a way to send the unmistakable message that she would kill him if he ever touched his grandchildren.

Carry and her husband stayed in the same little town as her parents for the next thirty years. Although Carry never told her husband about her childhood abuse, he later disclosed that he never felt comfortable around her father. He couldn't explain why, and Carry never disclosed the possible cause. By then her father had transformed into a respectable grandfather, and her husband and young son were never the wiser to the violent acts the man had once committed. Carry held her secret, not wanting to tarnish her son's image of his grandfather. However, her son was always under her watchful eye, ensuring his safety when he visited his maternal grandparents. Her father had three heart attacks, and he became a shell of the hateful, violent man he once was. Out of obligation, Carry helped her mother. Unfortunately, helping her mother meant helping her father, but she did so as the responsible, dutiful, oldest daughter. When her father finally died of cancer, it was a joyous day for Carry.

When Carry married, she threw herself into her own life of caring for her husband and son. As a married woman, her responsibilities were no longer to her parents and siblings. She developed a strong sense of purpose, and that purpose was to raise a strong and healthy son. It was a life that Carry loved. Although her past would cross her mind from time to time, she learned the valuable skill of remembering and then setting the memories aside so she could go on. As she told me, "You can let it destroy you, or you can move on." Her younger siblings never spoke of the horrific events, and as the years went by Carry began to wonder how much they even remembered. She had borne the brunt of the abuse, and it had stopped for them when they were fairly young.

Throughout Carry's marriage, she always had dogs. One of the most memorable was a wonderful deaf dog named Sally. Training a deaf dog was a challenge, but Carry's persistence and creativity paid off. Carry placed her throat on Sally's head so the dog could feel the vibrations of her words and understand that Carry was trying to communicate with her. She taught Sally to watch Carry's face, and she used sign language to teach the basic commands. Carry tapped her foot on the floor to get Sally's attention, and Sally could feel the vibrations of the garage door opening or the slam of the back door to know when her people were coming home. Carry loved her dog, and even agreed to a preschool teacher's request that she bring Sally to class to visit with the children. Although Sally was not the best with children (she had a history of playfully nipping people's fannies as they ran), Sally was a good sport, and thus she informally introduced Carry to the joy of animal-assisted activities.

In 1996, Carry's mother suffered a stroke. In addition, her mother developed Alzheimer's, which resulted in the need to transition her into a nursing home. The siblings decided to move their mother close to one of the other siblings, which was a relief to Carry. In 2004, Carry and her husband decided to move to Wyoming, where they had a retirement home. Even though Carry's husband had not yet retired, they decided it was time to make the move. Leaving Oklahoma behind was a relief to Carry. Although she had learned to manage her past well, all the painful memories were still associated with that little town, and moving to a new state provided a fresh start.

Sally had passed away at the age of fifteen, after living a long and productive life, and Carry had made up her mind that with her new start should come a new dog. She needed one that was good in the mountainous terrain in which they lived, so after extensive research, she chose a Saint Bernard. Ironically, the breeder almost didn't allow her to take the dog because she lived in the mountains. However, the breeder eventually decided the pup would have a good home with Carry, and she named her new puppy Maggie. (Carry laughed when she told me this part of the story since many of her friends often joke that they hope to be reincarnated as Carry's dog due to the love and attention she bestows on her pets.)

During their obedience classes at the local pet store, Maggie was immediately drawn to children. During one class the trainer couldn't help but mention that Maggie might be good as a therapy dog. Intrigued, Carry began to research the possibility. Unfortunately, she soon learned that there weren't any organized groups in her immediate area. After her initial thought of organizing a local chapter, she soon determined that was too much effort and resigned herself to making the two and a half hour drive to the nearest city to be a part of an already established group.

About then, Carry received the call she knew was coming. Her mother's condition had worsened, and she needed to go visit her in the nursing home and to support her siblings. Carry had come to dread these visits. Her mother's Alzheimer's had progressed to the point where she denied that Carry was even her daughter. Her mother blamed Carry for putting her in the nursing home, and her words were heavily laced with blame and hurtful comments. However, Carry needed to be there for her sister. Maggie was now a source of comfort and companionship for Carry, so she decided to take Maggie along to ease the stress of what lay ahead. To Carry's surprise, Maggie immediately disliked the nursing home. "It must be the odd smells," Carry thought to herself as she did her best to convince the hundred-pound Maggie that there was nothing to fear. However, as they approached her mother's room, Maggie body-blocked the doorway, making it clear that under no circumstances was Carry to enter. Carry's sister, who was standing by her mother's bed, looked up just in time to give Carry a perplexed expression as she witnessed dog and owner briefly hesitate at the doorway and then disappear down the corridor. It wasn't until they were safely on the other side of the locked doors of the nursing home unit that Maggie relaxed and returned to her sweet, laid-back disposition. It was then that Carry realized that Maggie's initial apprehension wasn't because of the smells at all. Maggie was painfully aware of Carry's conflicted feelings about her mother, and Maggie saw no need for Carry to subject herself to such an unpleasant encounter. Maggie had become Carry's protector; the one who helped her through the difficult emotions on the path toward healing.

Once Carry's mother passed away, her younger siblings began to contact her with questions about their childhood. They did remember horrific stories, and now found it comforting to verify remembered facts. For the first time in her adult life, Carry had someone to talk to about her past. With the airing of the memories came pain, but also came healing. She now knew it was time to tell her husband about her painful past. As the terrible memories came tumbling out, her husband now understood his discomfort around his father-in-law. The missing pieces had been found. Maggie had entered Carry's life at the very time that she needed her emotional support the most. During the most difficult times, Maggie would simply come over to Carry and rest her enormous head over her shoulder or on her chest in a doggy-style hug. Maggie was always there, and she seemed to show a different, more comforting side with Carry as compared with how she interacted with Carry's husband. With her husband, Maggie would transform into a hundred-pound puppy, her hindquarters swaying from side to side as she loped her way toward him and then gave a canine smile as she drove her two front paws into his lap. While Maggie showed her more playful side with her human dad, she was more snuggly and simply present with Carry. "She just kinda knows," Carry confided in me. Together they took long walks in the woods, Carry lost in her thoughts as she sorted out her past and Maggie always up for enjoying the sights and sounds of a forest romp.

Yet one of the most helpful ways that Maggie heals Carry's heart is in their work with children. Once a week, Carry makes the long drive into the city to work in an elementary school that specializes in educating children with profound disabilities. Many of the children are wheelchair-bound. Some cannot speak, and others cannot hear. Oxygen tanks and odd-looking apparatus are commonplace in this setting. Carry was quick to tell me that it is easier for her when she doesn't know the history, for it helps her just to be present. What a wonderful reminder that one's past does not define who one is today, nor who one can be tomorrow. She told me about a young boy, most likely about four years old, with Down Syndrome, who was terribly afraid of Maggie when they first met. His eyes became wide like saucers. He had never seen such a big dog! But, with time, he learned that Maggie was wonderfully friendly. During a recent visit to the school, Carry and Maggie walked into the hallway to find children playing on tricycles. As soon as this young boy saw Maggie, his face lit up with joy, a heartwarming smile spread across his face, and he pedaled as fast as his little legs could manage to Maggie. He then enjoyed some time petting Maggie, which ended with a high five to Carry.

"Volunteering really helps," Carry concluded. In doing so, she has found a way to give back to children and to be present for them even though adults were not present for her as a child. "They have it so much worse than me," she told me. It clearly gives her joy to reach out to these little ones with her big dog by her side. As we neared the end of our time together, she disclosed that her husband thought she should see a therapist. When I gently questioned why, she said it was simply because she had been through so much and her husband thought that surely she must need to talk to a professional. I smiled as I thought how perfectly Carry and Maggie's story illustrates the theme of this book. Carry had instinctively done everything a trained professional would ever advise—set clear limits around the abuser and keep others safe, understand that the abuse was not her fault, learn to set aside her emotions at times to allow herself to function, process and revisit the emotions/memories during appropriate times, talk with trusted confidants, reach out to others to keep her problems in perspective, and go on with her life. She was the textbook case of resiliency, and Maggie was the model therapy dog. Carry had already seen the best therapist of all—Maggie.

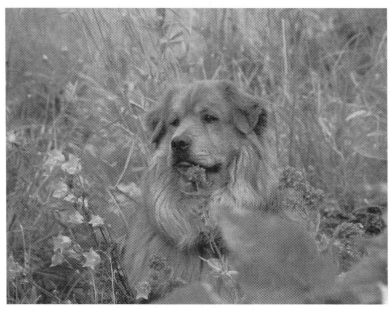

Molly
*Photo by Randy Oxley*

# Chapter Four
# Molly

*The dog lives for the day, the*
*hour, even the moment.*

—Robert Falcon Scott

My mornings usually begin in a very predictable way. I am not particularly a fan of early mornings, so my husband generally wakes and decides to begin his morning before I am willing to accept the impending day. He wakes without an alarm and does his best not to disturb me, but I am always awakened by the clang of the latches on Jasper's crate as Mark opens his gate. The resultant sounds are always the same—the rustling as Jasper bounds out of his crate, the canine groans ending with a high pitched squeak as Jasper does his morning stretch and yawn (I'm fairly certain that Mark joins in on this part of the routine as well, although I have not made the effort to open my eyes to know for sure), followed by a full, invigorating shake from head to tail, and lastly loving pats from Mark as they engage in their morning greeting. During this brief period, I quietly assess my position in bed, moving my face as needed and bracing for the next part of the routine. Mark can then be heard shuffling toward Rocky to unzip the flap on his large, soft-sided crate.

Now, Jasper is not a slow dog, so even early in the pre-dawn hours, he races from place to place, making it easy to track his location throughout the quiet house. I then hear the scramble of four paws around the perimeter of the king-sized bed that culminates in an exuberant pounce of his front paws on precisely the same position of the bed each morning. Before Jasper adopted this routine, that spot was where I usually rested my head as I enjoyed the remaining moments of sleep. However, after suffering a few painful, albeit unintended, scratches, I have adjusted my sleeping position in self-defense. Now Jasper lands close enough that I can feel the resounding thud of his forearms and paws and feel his warm breath without risking injury. Once Jasper has completed his predictable pounce, I join in the morning ritual, slowly bringing an arm out from under the toasty warm covers to give him a hug and moving my face close enough to receive a cherished wet whiskery kiss before he scurries off with his canine brother and "dad" for his morning trip out the basement door to do his business. Rocky can be heard trailing behind, happily panting with each step.

Just when I have drifted back to sleep, I am awakened once more by the sound of thunderous paws on the twenty-six stairs on the return journey, which is only broken by the sound of four paws struggling for traction as Jasper hits the first floor landing and does his best to gain the needed footing to make the sharp right turn on the hardwood flooring toward the second story. The tempo of the charging footsteps changes as Jasper bounds his way down the hallway and comes to a sudden halt right back beside the bed. He then rests his head on the edge of the bed for his final snuggle before he lies down and waits for my alarm clock to announce it's time to get up. Much slower, Rocky can be heard making his way into the bedroom, panting as though he was walking at one of his "faster" paces, and then rubbing up next to my side of the bed to benefit from any remaining petting that I am awake enough to offer. Content to receive his full morning greeting when I get up, he then lies down with a loud sigh and falls back asleep. It is a joyous way to be awakened.

Ask most dog lovers, and they will smile as they recall the sheer joy their dogs display each time their pets return to a room and see them. Dogs have a special way of lowering their heads and smiling in recognition, their tails wagging in a relaxed greeting, as they make a beeline toward their people. Their enthusiastic greeting remains the same even if it has only been minutes since the previous interaction. It is heartwarming. Such a simple gesture of love. One evening Rocky and I were giving a presentation about the human-animal bond with a colleague, when my human co-presenter spoke about the tremendous joy he received when his beloved pet would get up off her couch (yes, his dog sleeps on her own couch) after everyone else had gone to bed, to greet him at the door as he returned late at night from a hectic day. He then jokingly stated, "Even my wife won't do that!" These seemingly small acts of unconditional love, spontaneously offered by our dogs, are usually the things that warm our hearts the most. Precisely such a seemingly small canine interaction paved the way for Molly to enter the wonderful work of animal-assisted therapy. Here is her story.

Emily has always had dogs and known the special role they can play, but it wasn't until her mother suffered a sudden life-threatening heart attack that she really understood the healing powers dogs could offer to strangers. Her mother had been terribly worried by her sudden, deteriorating health. After a career in nursing, she understood too well the potentially devastating aftermath of various health conditions, such as stroke. Although she later learned she had not suffered a stroke and that her prognosis was good, the stress of illness and impending change was still weighing heavy on her mind. One day as Emily accompanied her mother walking the halls for the prescribed exercise, the IV pole alongside, they noticed a kind woman coming down the hospital hallway pulling a miniature cart that held a small papillon. This tiny dog was Emily's first introduction to the amazing work of therapy dogs. The wonderful dog had long silky white fur with patches of color over each eye; he had large, colored, butterfly-like ears. Emily's mother had always loved dogs, but she was partial to large dogs and had a tendency to be fairly derisive of small dogs. Given the circumstances, though, she welcomed the tiny dog and didn't seem to notice its stature. After thoroughly enjoying a visit with the therapy dog and his handler, Emily's mother happily chatted about how much this simple visit made her day, her face becoming notably brighter with each word. Gone momentarily were the worries and symbols of illness. Struck by the difference in her mother after such a short interaction with strangers, Emily made a mental note, but did nothing more.

According to Emily, four is the perfect number of household dogs. While she has had times during which she and her husband have had fewer than four, it just isn't right, Emily says with a twinkle in her eye. After enduring the difficult and sudden loss of her little beagle, Ellie, to congestive heart failure on Christmas day, she and her husband decided it was time to go to the local Humane Society to find another canine to join the family. Emily and her husband prefer to rescue dogs. Ellie had joined their family after following Emily home one snowy day. Emily's husband had come to accept that dogs just appeared—they were meant to be a part of their lives. True to this pattern and thinking it best to add another small dog to fill the hole left by Ellie, they had their hearts set on a wonderful little beagle mix who had been abandoned at the shelter and needed a good home. However, as they were walking toward the exit after committing to the tiny pup who needed to remain at the shelter for a few more days, a six-to nine-month-old, forty-five-pound, Newfoundland/chow mix puppy caught Emily's eye. The orange-red pup was in the cage on the far end; any further down the row, and they would not even have noticed her. She was incredibly mellow, and something about her made them rethink their decision. The pup had come to the Humane Society with a large black Newfoundland, most likely the little pup's father. Although it fleetingly crossed their mind to adopt both father and daughter to keep them together, it was more than they were willing to do. They already had a large shepherd/chow/akita mix who would not have tolerated another male in the home, regardless of the new dog's disposition. As Emily completed the necessary paperwork, she returned to find her husband and the new puppy comically sitting side by side on the bench in front of the Humane Society awaiting the journey home. The two looked as though they were posing for a picture for a brochure on behalf of the joys of dog adoption. Emily asked if her husband had invited the pup onto the bench, and he smiled, saying, "She just jumped up here!" They left the Humane Society that St. Patrick's Day weekend with the Newfoundland/chow mix, leaving the little beagle and the large Newfoundland behind. They named their new family member Molly in honor of her red hair and the holiday.

Molly was an incredibly easy dog right from the start. She was naturally calm, friendly, sensitive, and giving, with absolutely none of the disciplinary problems characteristic of puppies, such as chewing, accidents, or jumping onto people. Molly would politely sit on the couch and offer support, always sensitive to the needs of her new family. They realized how lucky they truly were to find such a remarkable dog. Emily soon thought to herself, "This is a dog who has to be shared!" It wasn't long before Emily remembered the tiny papillon from two years past and the tremendous impact he had on her mother during her darkest hours at the hospital. That was the answer! The only snag was that the hospital typically did not use dogs under the age of four or five; initially the administrators judged Molly to be too young for the program. But the trainer agreed to meet with Molly despite her young age and was immediately struck by her friendly, calm disposition. After Molly and Emily were tentatively accepted into a local hospital therapy dog program pending additional training, they completed a twelve-week obedience class (one that, as Emily quickly clarified to me, wasn't ever really needed due to Molly's exemplary behavior). They then completed an additional five weeks of intensive training to qualify officially to visit at the local hospital. Emily began researching national therapy dog programs in order to expand her work to other locations throughout the community, and she soon discovered the Wyoming-based program Therapy Dogs, Inc. After working with a local trainer for

Therapy Dogs, Inc., Emily and Molly were certified and ready to expand their volunteer work.

Working in hospital settings honed Molly's sensitivity to people. With time, Emily noticed that Molly found a way to indicate who truly needed her. With a gentle gesture of her paw, she motioned Emily toward the person who needed her most. In addition, Molly had a propensity to snuggle with almost anyone she met in the hallways. Her specialty soon became oncology. When she sensed a patient had a special need, she would lift her paw toward the person and then gently set her paw on his/her bed. Molly also perfected the ability to ensure that each person in a room received a visit; moving purposefully from person to person until each could benefit from stroking her soft fur or enjoying a snuggle. She would lovingly rest her head gently on patients' laps or on their beds while they petted her; a trait her patients found endearing.

After becoming comfortable working in various settings throughout the local hospitals, Emily made a proposal to the local hospice care to develop a therapy dog program. They enthusiastically accepted her proposal, and Molly became the first therapy dog in the hospice system in that area. One of Molly's first patients was an elderly gentleman who was seriously depressed, but refusing visits from anyone other than his nurse. He was not a "dog person," but following some gentle prodding from his nurse, he agreed to a trial visit from Molly. Upon meeting Molly, he became immediately enamored with her and eagerly waited for their visits, the apartment door left open and a bowl of water waiting each week. Pictures of Molly became part of the man's décor, and the long chats he enjoyed with Emily as he spent hours petting Molly were the highlight of his week.

In addition, Molly and Emily began working with a wonderful program that provided services to children who had lost a parent and were struggling with grief. Each child enjoyed a special session with Molly and a therapist with complete freedom to talk about anything they chose. They could even say nothing at all. Molly and Emily loved the hospice and grief work, but Emily decided it was becoming too draining when her own mother became ill and passed away, so they went on hiatus. The programs continue without Molly, with many other dogs carrying on the work Emily and Molly started. As Emily told me about their work in hospice, she commented that it might be time to return now that she has had time to grieve her mother's passing. In the interim, Emily decided to volunteer at a local elementary school to assist children who were having difficulty with their reading. This is where I first met Emily and Molly.

It was a beautiful late winter day as I parked my car and watched for a dog who met the description of an "orange newfie." The sun was shining brightly, making it feel much warmer than the actual temperature. A car pulled into the elementary school parking lot, and a large orange head poked out of the back window and then retreated quickly back inside as the driver maneuvered the car into a parking space. Although I wasn't able to get a good look at the dog's features, I surmised, "That has to be them." As I grabbed my keys and began walking toward them, I saw a second orange dog on the left, walking with a kind-looking older woman. Surprised to see two identically colored dogs in the same location, I began to look beyond the dog's color to match the description. Molly's Newfoundland characteristics made her easy to spot—her silky, heavy coat, soft eyes, and droopy lower lips. She was wearing a bright red vest with a patch on one side that read, "Paws to Listen," and a second patch on her back that read, "Molly." After brief introductions, Emily took Molly off the grassy area to a patch of weeds and untamed foliage where Molly quickly did her business before we entered the elementary school. "Molly won't pee on grass," Emily explained. Living in the foothills of the Rocky Mountains, Molly isn't use to grass since park-like grass is not a part of the mountainous terrain.

As we entered the elementary school, one of the office staff members exclaimed, "Who's there? Is that my Molly?" as she came around the glass partition to visit with the therapy dog. As Emily signed our names on the visitor list, the staff member enjoyed a visit with Molly, chatting away about her own dogs and about how much she enjoyed Molly's weekly visits. From a distance, two young students pointed and whispered in excited tones before scurrying into a nearby classroom. With visitor badges in place, we made our way down the hallway, Molly's tail gently wagging as she led the way to the waiting classroom.

Upon entering the colorful classroom, we were immediately greeted by Lisa, "Teacher Extraordinaire," as Emily described her with a smile. Lisa was a young, warm, inviting woman, who quickly demonstrated her ability to multitask as two children entered the room simultaneously, both in need of direction. She greeted them both by name and quickly encouraged them each to pick a book to read to Molly. She then seamlessly turned, finished her welcome, and directed Emily to take Molly to "Molly Land" (the term lovingly assigned to the far corner of the room). Molly Land consisted of a large pink flannel blanket detailed with playful ladybugs laid across the tile floor. Bookcases provided a tiny alcove and gave the sense of privacy. I took a seat in one of the tiny chairs by a nearby table, hoping to be able to quietly observe Molly and Emily in their element; Molly was quickly surrounded by children holding books, excited to demonstrate their reading skills.

It had been years since I had set foot in an elementary school classroom, and I was surprised by all the familiar sights. Every inch of wall space seemed to be used skillfully, with large poster boards listing class expectations and lessons in both English and Spanish. All were handwritten in colorful markers and in perfect printing. The colorful classroom had a lived-in organized-cluttered feel with bookshelves and tables teeming with books, papers, and other implements of learning. Several other children were gathered in another corner of the classroom, already quietly reading to Murphy, the other orange dog I had seen arriving earlier. Emily quickly welcomed the children as they came to read to Molly. She began by asking the children if they were going to read in English or Spanish, and skillfully demonstrated her bilingual abilities as she followed along, supportively coaching each child in whatever language chosen. Some children read alone, while others read a book together; some alternating pages while others read in unison. Once a book was completed, the children eagerly picked out a page of stickers from Emily's extensive collection; Emily spoke the names of the sticker characters in both English and Spanish to assist the children in finding the perfect page. It wasn't long before it was clear that puppies, kittens, Chihuahuas, and Curious George stickers were among the most popular.

As Emily was happily absorbed in listening to the reading child, waiting children petted and hugged Molly as she patiently sat taking in the scene. Others showed Molly bookmarks they had received after reading to Murphy, and Molly appreciatively sniffed each one. Molly looked at me on occasion with her soft loving eyes and her mouth in her characteristic doggy smile that revealed her chow-like blue-black tongue. She seemed to be enjoying the attention and hoping I was dutifully noting it all down. Throughout the hour, children continued to come to the classroom as those who had already read to each dog disappeared into the hallway. Each new child was quickly noticed by "Miss Lisa," and she helped each one prepare to read to Molly. She would say, "That one is too easy! Pick another book," or, "I would like you to practice this one to read to Molly next week. Don't you think she would like that one?"

During a brief break, Emily warned, "There may be another deluge of children. I don't know where they come from; they just appear!" True to her words, another wave of children soon appeared, and the reading continued as Miss Lisa made note of each and every child to ensure each need was addressed.

Amongst the well-controlled chaos, a young boy named Jose

sat patiently on the floor beside Molly, waiting for his turn to read. He silently stroked Molly's soft fur and gave her multiple hugs. Molly responded by lifting her head to expose her neck so he could better reach the soft fur on her neck and chest for petting. It was touching to see such a tender moment between the dog and young boy. Jose and Molly clearly knew each other well and cherished this time together. When his turn came, he opened his book, and clearly did his best to read the assigned portion of *Wild, Wild Wolves*. After many minutes, Miss Lisa came over and noticed that, in his eagerness to read to Molly, Jose had read past the part she had assigned. She told him it was time to wrap up his reading time. Disappointed, he shut the book, clearly sad his time was over. Emily gently prodded Molly to move off the stickers so Jose could pick a reward for a job well done. Jose hugged and snuggled with Molly as he perused the available stickers.

Near the end of the reading time, a young child came in the room with a woman, both speaking Spanish in hushed tones. The woman pointed to Murphy as she spoke softly to the child and then to Molly as the child remained in close proximity. They then took a seat at the table across from Molly. They continued to speak in hushed tones as Molly dutifully lay beside Emily and the child reading. Then as quietly as they came, they stood up, spoke softly to Lisa, and left.

As the crowd of children gradually dwindled, Lisa came over to tell us that she was not expecting any additional children for the day. Emily finished up with the remaining children, and soon only the adults and therapy dogs remained. As Emily began to collect her things, I asked Lisa what difference Molly has made for her students. And then, to my surprise, she became quite emotional, and tears began to form in her eyes as she spoke about her beloved students. While I had noted from the beginning that she was a very conscientious teacher, I had somehow neglected to see the true depth of emotion she felt for these children. Then she spoke about the young boy, Jose. She told me how much he loves Molly and "needs her unconditional love." She went on to say that she uses Molly as a reward for good choices since Jose has Attention Deficit Hyperactivity Disorder and has been in trouble. She then proudly told me how much his reading and behaviors have improved as a result of reading to and loving Molly. A second child who struggles with dyslexia now writes stories about Molly in both English and Spanish. She came to Lisa reading at a kindergarten level, but thanks to this program now reads at a second-grade level. Most of the children in the program used to be afraid of dogs, she explained, similar to the child I had witnessed who just sat quietly with the woman at the table near the end of the reading session. With time, each learned how wonderful a dog could be. Now they know "the dogs are here to help."

As we said our good-byes to Lisa, two girls stood waiting to walk Molly down the hall. It was a touching little caravan down the hallway as Molly led the way with her tail wagging proudly; a young girl on each side, each holding the leash as Emily gently reassured Molly that she was truly the one in charge of the procession. As the children said their good-byes, Emily and I sat down for some time to chat. It was then that I truly discovered how much their work together had changed Emily.

Emily had clearly put some thought into this subject in anticipation of my questions, and she quickly rattled off many ways she was different because of Molly—able to meet people where they are, able to communicate better, able to be more accepting of everyone, more patient, able to put aside assumptions, able to better think and act on her feet, etc. As she was describing examples of each of these, she began to speak about the greatest lesson that was intertwined amongst them all. She mentioned all the small acts of kindness that Molly does each day, all the simple little things that would easily go unrecognized if one weren't watching carefully. The wag of her tail, the offer of her paw, her look of happy recognition, her very presence during a difficult moment—all of these tiny acts serve an important role in making an enormous difference in someone's life. But the most significant difference that Molly has made to Emily, she said, was that the human half of the team now does her best to offer such simply acts of kindness as well—opening a door for someone, allowing someone to step ahead of her in the line at the grocery store, offering a smile or a kind word. Each act alone may not seem like much, but she has learned from Molly that it doesn't take much to make someone's day. Her face lit up as she told me how grateful people have been for her small gestures. I could tell these small acts made her day as well.

Dogs are experts at bringing smiles to our faces. Their very presence can make our day. These seemingly small acts of unconditional love that our dogs do spontaneously are the very acts that warm our hearts the most. It only stands to reason that the same could be said of small acts of unconditional love done by humans to other humans. Is it any surprise that it would take a loving, big orange newfie to teach us such a wonderful lesson?

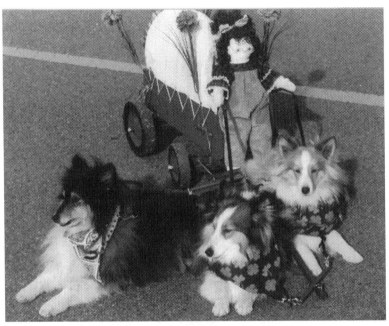

Dinkie with His Wild West Buddies
*Photo by Timme C. Wild*

# Chapter Five
# The Wild West Shelties

*To fear love is to fear life, and
those who fear life are already
three parts dead.*

—Bertrand Russell

When we fall in love we rarely put much thought into how the story will end. It's probably for the best, for as long as we live on this fragile planet, one is destined to die before the other. Some of the most touching love stories tell how the surviving partner, devastated by the loss of a soul mate, struggles to find a reason to carry on despite the gut-wrenching hole that will forever remain in his or her heart. Despite the knowledge that loss and pain are the inevitable, we continue to fall in love, somehow remembering the basic truth that love is worth the risk of pain. No where is this impending loss more true than when a human loves a dog. Given the difference in life expectancy, the outcome is easily predicted. One might even venture to wonder if that is by design. What better way for humans to begin to learn the lessons of old age, pain, and loss than through the lessons and examples of our canine friends? We have two choices—either to enjoy each moment we are given and then embrace and prepare for the inevitable, or to harden our hearts and become angry and bitter that it always ends in heartache and death. Our pets lead by example by thoroughly enjoying each and every moment they are given, never thinking of what could have been or what they wish they had.

One of the hardest decisions therapy dog handlers ever have to make is when it is time to say good-bye to their beloved partner and friend. When is it best to let nature take its course, and when is it more humane to step in and stop the suffering? Our therapy dogs depend on us for protection and love, and this decision is the ultimate in both of these all-important traits. It is an immensely personal decision, and one in which others can only offer words of comfort, but never advice. It was at such a fork in the road that I sat down with Maggie Wild to hear all about her beloved Dinkie. Dinkie was not present at this meeting, for his health was failing, but his younger brother Corky eagerly came in his stead. Maggie carefully spread Corky's blanket on the couch between us and then lifted him onto his spot. He provided just the comfort and distraction that we both needed as we both intermittently stroked his thick fur as we chatted for the next hour and a half.

I was happy to have received the e-mail from Maggie offering Dinkie's story, for I remembered him well. He was an adorable tri-colored, seventeen-pound sheltie that helped out with my own dogs' therapy exam by confidently walking by to test my collies' ability to ignore a "neutral dog." It was always a part of the exam I dreaded, for my pups were always eager to play, chase, or otherwise engage in canine fun despite the seriousness of the examination. While I was tense and determined to pass the test with flying colors, my pups had no such worries—they were just themselves, enjoying every moment and looking for fun. Dinkie, on the other hand, was the consummate professional as he strolled by, seemingly oblivious to his surroundings. He was the dog to emulate. Today I was eager to hear all about this little dynamo, but I was not prepared to learn the worst. At thirteen years of age, Dinkie was losing his second bout with Cushing's Disease, and he had significant mobility problems due to a bad back knee. Maggie said that she wasn't sure how much pain he was in, but they were doing all they could for him. I could see the anguish in Maggie's eyes as she began to talk about her little buddy's pain. It was only when she started to talk about his life and the joy he brought to her and others that her eyes began to sparkle. I could tell she knew that the joy Dinkie's life had brought was going to help her through the pain soon to come. Here is Dinkie's story.

Dinkie started his life off on the wrong paw, so to speak. He had been returned to his original breeder on two different occasions by families who thought he was the perfect dog for them. The relationships started off well, but Dinkie soon found himself back to square one, looking for a forever home. Dinkie, it seemed, could not do anything right. However, for Dinkie, the third try was a charm, and he came to live with Maggie and her husband, Timme. Maggie never bothered to ask why he had been returned by others on those two occasions. It just didn't matter to her. Although Maggie had loved dogs all her life and always envisioned herself having her own shelties some day, she happened to marry a kind man who was terrified of dogs. He had been bitten on four or five occasions throughout his life, and trusting another canine was not something he was eager to try. When he came home one day from out-of-state travel, he found that Maggie had adopted the one-and-a-half-year-old Dinkie. Initially, Dinkie would have nothing to do with Timme, but after two weeks Dinkie started following him through the house. Before long Timme was taking Dinkie for walks, and the rest is history. That was probably the first miracle that Dinkie performed in his life as a therapy dog. Even skilled therapists would have been proud of Dinkie's ability to heal a deep-seated fear in such a short period of time.

Dinkie was not the stereotypical sheltie. He was always quiet, and not much would get him riled up. It was even a good three months before they ever heard him bark. He was never one to play or chase a ball. (This could be why he was returned, Maggie surmised. He wouldn't be a good dog for someone who wanted to play.) He could best be described as a dignified gentleman. Playing was beneath him; sitting on the roof of the house overlooking his property was more his style, much to the shock of his new parents. Maggie reminisced that she thought her neighbor was terribly mistaken when he first told her that Dinkie was spotted on the roof of the house. She later learned that Dinkie was me-thodically jumping on the top of his crate on the back deck, then onto the deck railing, and finally walking up the sloped roof to his vantage point.

Approximately a year later, Maggie decided it was time to add another sheltie to the family. That sheltie was a little mahogany sable puppy named Aspen. Soon after, Maggie said she was stop-ping traffic as drivers turned to watch as she walked the two pups proudly down the road. She was quick to understand that these two little dogs had quite a special gift, and true to her own kind heart, she began to search for a way to share them with others. She started by having the pups drag a gallon milk jug around the neighborhood to help them become comfortable with something dragging and making noise behind them. This progressed to a little red Radio Flyer wagon and eventually to a pioneer-style wagon that was specially designed and built just for them. Before long they were well known on the parade circuit as the "Wild West Shelties." Both dogs loved the attention, and Maggie had found a special way to bring smiles to the faces of children and adults alike as she traveled throughout the country sharing her dogs' special talents.

As time passed and Dinkie began to age, she decided she needed another way to share Dinkie's gifts with others. She ad-opted a third sheltie (the sweet-natured sable-and-white puppy she named Corky). Corky soon took over Dinkie's position pull-ing the covered wagon in parades, and Dinkie began to learn about the world of being a therapy dog. Although Dinkie had a wonderful mellow, easygoing personality, Maggie later learned that her dog trainer never thought he would make it as a therapy dog. He just didn't show any interest in the work, which is a requirement in order to ensure the dog's well-being. What the trainer didn't realize is that Dinkie didn't show *any* outward inter-est in *anything*, but Maggie knew his heart and she pushed on despite failing the therapy dog test multiple times. Dinkie didn't like being crowded by others (an important element of the test). Eventually Maggie began to understand that the handler must do the learning in these settings to protect the therapy dog and ensure an enjoyable interaction for all, and she soon mastered the ability to effectively manage these situations. They then passed the test and began visiting clients in a variety of settings.

Dinkie was the perfect size and temperament to be placed on a hospital towel on or beside sick patients. Because of his tiny size, he was even able to visit despite limited space and the complexity of equipment found in hospitals settings. Dinkie was intuitive and seemed to sense the importance of remaining perfectly still and enjoying the touch of the patient. At times he just sat with patients who were unconscious, seemingly unaware of his presence, as Maggie helped the patient stroke Dinkie's soft fur. On one occasion, Maggie brought Dinkie into the room to visit a patient only to learn that the patient and his family spoke only a little English. Despite the language barrier, it became clear that the patient wanted a visit, so Maggie quickly placed Dinkie on a hospital towel on the patient's chest. Before Dinkie's visit, the man's face was tense and anxious, but soon his hands were buried deep in Dinkie's fur, his eyes tightly shut. The man never spoke or opened his eyes, only quietly enjoyed Dinkie's presence. Over the course of that visit, the man's facial expression changed from tense and anxious to peaceful and serene. His wife later expressed her gratitude for the visit, and as they left the nurse disclosed to Maggie that the man was a retired veterinarian from Russia.

After one such visit Maggie and Dinkie were walking down the hospital hallway. Maggie sensed that Dinkie was not yet ready to go home, so they headed for the Intensive Care Unit waiting room to continue to visit. As they approached, Maggie saw a gentleman leaning against the wall who appeared to have a heavy heart. After their visits in the waiting room they returned the same way and again saw this man, now sitting alone. Maggie decided to engage him in a conversation and offer a visit from

Dinkie. The man gratefully accepted, and soon Dinkie was sitting on his special blanket on the gentleman's lap; the man was clearly enjoying Dinkie's presence. The story soon unfolded. The gentleman was a physician and his professional partner was extremely ill and would likely never practice medicine again. His partner's parents were also in the waiting room, and were clearly distraught. After a significant amount of time had passed, the physician told Maggie and his partner's parents that his heart was no longer racing as it had been before the visit, and that he felt a sense of calm that previously seemed unimaginable given the stressfulness of his circumstances.

That was Dinkie's special gift, this ability to quietly be while making a tremendous impact on those whom he visited. Now Corky was following in those tiny footsteps and continuing Dinkie's therapy dog legacy. Corky patiently allowed me to run my fingers through his soft fur and fiddle with his paws as I listened to Dinkie's story. I could just imagine how comforting this would be to one who is sick. It was easy to tell what a difference Dinkie had made for others, and even for Maggie's husband. Maggie was quick to tell me how much her husband now loves dogs; he even stops people on the street to meet their dogs. He even has been known to invite all three pups onto the bed on Saturday mornings for a few moments of play and snuggle time. Dinkie showed Timme the joy that can only come from loving a dog. But how about Maggie? She had always known how wonderful dogs could be. How had Dinkie changed her?

One of the things that struck me about Maggie was that she described herself as shy. This label seemed in marked contrast to the warm, inviting person who quickly rose in greeting as I entered the nursing home where we had agreed to meet. As my eyes met hers, I instantly felt welcome. Throughout our time together, those passing through the lobby smiled, waved, or came over for a quick hello from Maggie and her canine buddy, Corky. None of this seemed characteristic of a shy person. She later went on to explain that being with her dogs makes it possible for her to do or say what's in her heart. They free her from her shyness, and allow her to share her life with complete strangers. Through the dogs she is able to show compassion and love for her fellow humans and be the kind of person she believes she is meant to be. It was through recognizing that her dogs have a very special gift that Maggie found her own gift, and it became an avenue for her love to shine to others. As she spoke about the importance of learning how to recognize a dog's unique talent and how one must then "plug the dog into their talent," it became clear that Maggie had been plugged into her own very special talent through the love of her dogs.

As our time grew to a close, my thoughts again were on Dinkie, now frail and in ill health. Maggie asked if I had ever had to make the very painful decision to euthanize a cherished pet. I had. She said that she thought it was time for her beloved Dinkie to breathe his last breath, but it was now her husband, Timme, who was not yet ready to say good-bye. Are any of us ever truly ready to say good-bye? I tried to leave her with words of comfort, but I knew in my heart that there really are none to be given. The pain of losing one that you love is an unfortunate part of this life, but it is the necessary price of the joy that loving brings. It is the signal to the end of a love story that was well worth living and sharing. Good-bye, dear Dinkie.[3]

---

3  On Thursday, September 6, 2007, Dinkie breathed his last breath. When I spoke with Maggie shortly after, she told me through her tears, "It was for the best." It was time for them to part. Maggie and Timme later adopted another sheltie pup who is bringing laughter and smiles to the home.

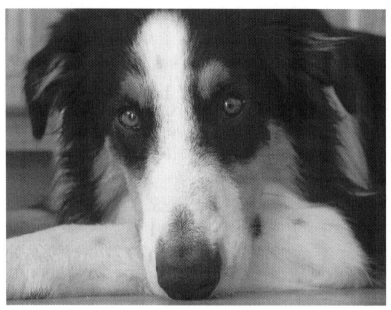

Jasper
*Photo by Teri Pichot*

# Chapter Six
# Jasper

*Properly trained, a man [or
woman] can be a dog's best
friend.*

—Corey Ford

Jasper was what some would call an impulse buy. Although the idea of getting another dog to train as a second therapy dog and family pet had intermittently crossed my mind, my husband and I had not made the final decision, nor were we officially looking for the perfect dog. Granted, I had been perusing Internet sites for available rough coat collie puppies (something that I continue to do to this day as a harmless form of window shopping), but not with the true intention of falling in love and bringing one into our family right then. We were just beginning to recover from two hectic years of socializing and training our first collie, Rocky. Rocky was finally maturing into an adult dog who required less supervision, which allowed for more time for non-dog related activities. Overall, Rocky had been an easy dog to train. He was intelligent, enjoyed the dog school scene, and loved to be with people. He was the first dog whom I took the time to truly understand and formally train, and this process introduced me to the wonderful world of animal-assisted therapy. I was intrigued by the idea that a trained dog could engage people of all ages and cultures, and I loved the genuineness he brought out in me and everyone else around him. He had the gift of lighting up a room and finding the deeply hidden smile in the grumpiest person. He even had inspired me to write a book about the amazing work that Rocky did at a local health department. As the months passed, he perfected the ability to sleep for hours at my feet while

I typed away at the keyboard. This quiet togetherness is one of the things I love most about having a dog.

But one sunny September day I found myself looking at the unexpected—a four-month-old tri-color rough coat collie puppy advertised on the Pueblo Collie Rescue Web site. The description stated that he was born in a Kansas shelter after his pregnant mother was found wandering the streets. Finding a puppy through a rescue was rare, but especially one so young and yet free of any history of horrific abuse or neglect. Despite my better judgment I excitedly told my husband, Mark, about my find. Discovering a puppy who didn't come with a fear of people from being mistreated was invaluable in my long-term goal of training him for therapy dog work. While no dog ever comes with a guarantee that he will be able to excel at therapy work, a dog free from abuse and neglect increases the odds. This was all part of my argument. Looking back on that day, I realize Mark was just humoring me when he told me to call the phone number and get more information. While he was open to the idea of a second dog someday soon, as a rule he is not one to feel comfortable with impromptu decisions. To my surprise, I received a return phone call within fifteen minutes despite it being a Sunday afternoon. The kind voice encouraged us to make the two and a half hour drive south to Pueblo that very day to meet little Jasper and see if he would make a good addition to our family. It was then that Mark began to express his concern about adding a second dog to our family, but I quickly assured him that we were "just looking" and would only bring the pup home if we both agreed he was a perfect fit. It is in reminiscing upon conversations such as the one that occurred that day that I began to truly appreciate how well my husband knows me. True to his predictions, the pup came home with us that day despite his reservations.

Our first glimpse of Jasper was through his foster mom's screen door. An excited Jasper was jumping and barking enthusiastically as we made our way up the walkway. He was nothing like our calm and gentle Rocky! Used to Rocky's well-mannered, easy-going nature, we were initially taken aback by Jasper' antics. He was impossible to hold as he frantically tried to lick my face, squirming as his entire hindquarters wagged. Then I got my first glimpse at his malformed right ear. It was comically laying across the top of his head like a bad toupee. "We tacked it down with some fabric glue to try to tame it," his foster mom quickly volunteered. "I told him we had to do something or all the other dogs were going to make fun of him," she added with a smile. The wayward ear, coupled with his exuberance, were not what we had anticipated in our dream pup, but Jasper's innocent doggy smile had a way of insisting that we give him a chance. Sensing our apprehension, our host quickly encouraged us to take Jasper for a walk with Rocky to get to know him better. Rocky was not amused, and he kept a close eye on the young pup. He seemed annoyed to have to share a cherished walk with such an unruly young canine, and he expressed his displeasure through occasional vocal canine corrections warning the pup to pay attention and stop crashing into him. I walked the genteel Rocky, while Mark wrestled with the crazed Jasper.

Within a few hours, we were on our way home with Jasper lying peacefully on my lap and Rocky seething in the back seat. I knew that bringing a little brother into Rocky's life would be an adjustment, but I was woefully unprepared for what lay ahead. Rocky had a good life; he had a plethora of rawhides and toys, and we doted on him each time he entered the room. He was not prepared to share this life with a stray who had not been part of the family plan even twenty-four hours earlier. As we opened the kitchen door, exhausted from the trip, the battle began. Rocky rushed Jasper, pinning him under the kitchen cabinet and verbally assaulting him for what seemed like an eternity. Rocky's barking was deafening, and poor Jasper continued to be the target of these canine-style lectures each time he moved. Gone was our easy-going Rocky as he made it clear to the newcomer that everything was his and nothing was up for grabs. It was then that I conceded that Mark was right; bringing Jasper home was a mistake. I agreed to consider returning him to Pueblo should a phone call to Rocky's dog trainer, Ashley, the next morning fail to provide much-needed guidance.

Exhausted, we took the dogs outside to do their business, planning to then put Jasper in a crate to sleep so Rocky would calm down and let us all rest. Then, to our amazement, the unexpected happened. Rocky's tone suddenly changed to a playful "woof" as he went down on his front elbows in the grass and his tail wagged happily in the air in a canine invitation to play. Jasper, initially as surprised by Rocky's change in demeanor as we were, then reciprocated with a play bow of his own, followed by an exuberant game of catch-me-if-you-can as both dogs romped in the moonlight. Relieved by the happy sight, we watched in amazement as the dogs wrestled and played like they were long-lost friends. "Maybe it wasn't such a bad idea," Mark said. After enjoying the peace for a while, we called the boys into the house only to have Rocky resume his bullying tactics as he continued to make sure the newcomer knew not to touch his things or chew on his rawhides. Jasper cried himself to sleep that night in his crate on one side of our bed while Rocky growled in low, quiet tones in response to Jasper's pitiful wails on the other side. It was a long night for us all.

As I spoke with Ashley the following morning, I found a glimmer of hope. She explained that Rocky's behavior was normal as an older, wiser dog setting limits and giving direction to a new pup, and that I had a lot of work ahead of me to reassure Rocky that Jasper was not a threat. Likewise, Jasper had a lot to learn about being respectful of his elders. She gave clear instructions regarding how to work with each dog and how to assist the boys in eventually establishing a peaceful pack. I was becoming painfully aware of how little I knew about canine culture and how steep my learning curve was going to be over the next year.

Relieved with the newfound information, I began implementing the prescribed structured regiment with good success. Mark came home for lunch, and we decided to make it an afternoon at the neighborhood park. With the picnic basket packed and both dogs in tow, we headed out across the manicured park lawns to our favorite spot. It was near the edge of the park, but with ample view of other park goers. Rocky and Jasper were acting the part of peaceful brothers enjoying the beautiful sunny day. With sandwiches in hand and leashes loosely fastened around the collapsible picnic chair to keep tabs on the pups while leaving our hands free for eating, we were just starting to enjoy our lunch when it happened. A gentleman was playing Frisbee with his dog across the park—a normal occurrence at a public park. Suddenly Jasper lunged, barking frantically and almost toppling Mark's chair in the rush of movement and noise. Mark's sandwich went flying as he struggled to manage the out-of-control Jasper. Sure that something horrible was underway, Rocky joined the ruckus, barking in support of Jasper; ignorant of the true cause of the uproar. Embarrassed, we regained control of our dogs, scolded Jasper appropriately, and settled in to resume our lunch. No sooner than we were seated, it all began again. The gentleman smirked in our direction and continued to play with his dog. He appeared to enjoy the entertainment factor as he seemed to instigate the ruckus for sport. After three or four episodes of this madness, Mark and I concluded that a peaceful lunch just wasn't possible. Jasper was now inconsolable at being only a spectator of the Frisbee game and was wailing as if he was being beaten. The man with the Frisbee yelled, "Why don't you train your dogs!" Now, I would like to say this story ended with Mark and me smiling sweetly, packing our bags, and inconspicuously leaving the park. Unfortunately, that just would not be true. Regrettably, a few choice words were exchanged, and we left in a huff; muttering under our breath that he had no idea the hours and money we had invested into Rocky's training. "He was a therapy dog, no less! Train our dogs!" How dare he think we were the kind of dog owners that neglect to provide our dogs with adequate training? Jasper was a puppy! What did he expect? Little did I know that this scene would become a regular part of our public life for the next three years. Maybe it is good I didn't know it then. I'm not sure I would have been so willing to invest the time and energy into the little guy had I known then what I know now.

In many ways, I have lived a privileged life. While my family struggled financially when I was a child, they strongly valued education and learning. This resulted in a plethora of individual attention that nurtured my innate abilities. As a result, many things just come naturally to me. I have always been very good with academics, and I have always been able to organize and understand both concepts and tasks. I naturally lean toward academics, creative arts, and other indoor activities. This has resulted in me being reasonably successful in most jobs and undertakings. When I have needed to work hard to understand or develop a challenging skill, I have been able to do so primarily in a private setting; only demonstrating the skill once it has been fully refined. The things in which I don't succeed, I have found a way to avoid—such as athletics, unstructured social settings, and more physical activities. This early knack to self-select into successful areas has served me well, but it has also left me woefully unprepared for public failure or humiliation.

Becoming a psychotherapist was something that fit my skill-set well. It is a profession that requires the ability to quickly understand sometimes complex or abstract concepts, yet benefits from a creative ear that can match research and concepts with each unique human being. Working with Rocky in this field was a natural extension of this purposeful creativity. The field of animal-assisted therapy was founded upon researched concepts, yet the spontaneity of the inclusion of a dog added the creative element that held my interest. While I stumbled into the field of animal-assisted therapy through my initial plans to simply teach my family pet some household manners, I found the basic constructs of dog training similar to the behavioral techniques for humans I had learned in school. These similarities, combined with my early success training Rocky, gave me what I now recognize as an inflated sense of confidence in my dog training abilities.

After signing Jasper up for the next series of puppy kindergarten classes, I decided to teach him the fundamentals to get a head start. I had come to enjoy the group classes, for they gave the needed information and environment for socialization while providing the opportunity to learn and practice the skills in the privacy of my own home each week. While the classes would require Jasper and me to perform our tasks in a group setting, it was entirely up to me how prepared we were each week. Given my prior experience with Rocky in these classes, I already had the basic knowledge, so I was determined to get started. Jasper was clearly a very smart dog, and he readily learned the basic commands: sit, down, stay, etc. Unlike Rocky, Jasper loves to please and immediately demonstrated an eagerness to do anything I asked once he understood the task. Jasper has an intensity about him. He plays and works with uncanny focus and gusto. By the date of our first class, Jasper was a star pupil. As the other kindergarteners struggled to comprehend what their human partners where asking of them, Jasper quickly knocked off multiple sits, always looking up to me with his characteristic "What's next?" expression.

With puppy school going so well and Rocky and Jasper gradually building a brotherly relationship, I decided to take my new little puppy for a drive to my favorite park for a walk. While not close to our house, it is the ideal setting for basic socialization, for it is well known in the Denver area for dog walkers, bikers, skaters, and all sorts of outdoor activities. It has various paved walkways and a dirt path that circles its perimeter, making it the ideal place for all outdoor enthusiasts. Eager to embark on our day's activities, Jasper and I headed out. It was a warm day, so shorts and sandals were the appropriate attire for me, and a Snoot Loop (similar to a Gentle Leader) was the equipment of choice for Jasper as the plan was to work on loose lead walking. I casually slung a bag full of water bottles, poop bags, and treats over my shoulder as I leashed up my little friend. It felt good to be out in the sunshine, being part of the community.

As we walked from our parked car to the main path, Jasper spotted a dog calmly walking with its owner several yards away, and he spontaneously transformed into the barking, snarling beast that I had only met that first day on our picnic from hell. Startled, I surmised it simply must be that I did not have a treat in hand and was not in training mode. Braving the concerned looks from passersby, I regrouped, regained Jasper's attention, and started out again, only to have Jasper dissolve into a deluge of lunging and barking at the very next dog he saw. Fellow park-goers pulled their children and pets close and widened their distance as I wrestled to regain control of the very loud and thrashing Jasper. Utterly humiliated and out of breath from the struggle, I eyed a spot under a tree, erroneously thinking that sitting with Jasper would be more manageable than walking. Clearly in better shape than I and overly stimulated by the surroundings, Jasper continued his antics on the way to the designated spot. I sat down and reeled him in like a fish. I then held his head in an effort to force his focus from others onto me, as he immediately succeeded in slithering out of my grasp to bark and lunge at onlookers once again. After exerting my last bit of energy, I finally was able to lift him up onto my lap, only to loosen my grip in response to searing pain as his back paws raked across my thigh in the flailing that ensued. Throughout the ordeal, Jasper was making a painful wail that sounded as though it came deep from within his toes and could only be the result of excruciating agony. The onlookers who were not terrified stopped to gawk, apparently wondering how to intervene, believing I must be abusing the poor, helpless puppy. "He's fine!" I yelled angrily, desperate for the stimulation and my own humiliation to diminish. Jasper gave one more wail as if begging them to rush over and save him. Thankfully, they just shook their heads and moved on.

Gone was my vision of a peaceful walk in the park with my new puppy. My only hope was to somehow make it back to my car, which now seemed miles away. With my leg bleeding and throbbing from the scratches and my pride completely shattered, we made a run for it. Jasper barked and scrambled as I pulled him backwards toward the car in an ungraceful spectacle. I was past all thoughts of training; I was in survival mode with the car as the only refuge. Once there, I buckled the sad Jasper into the back seat. He had transformed back into the sweet, loving pup and looked up at me as if asking, "What happened to our walk?" In the driver's seat at last, I sat motionless as tears began to well up. The scratches on my thigh were blending with forming bruises to create a large comet-like pattern. How could such a sweet little puppy cause such havoc?

Once home, Mark was in disbelief at my story. It wasn't until later outings during which Jasper exhibited similar behavior that Mark truly understood the gravity of the training issues. Ashley gave helpful suggestions and support. She reassured us that Jasper was not an aggressive dog. He simply had not learned to manage his emotions when his prey drive was triggered. She instructed us to step on his leash and ignore him, only letting him continue his walk once he regained his composure. She later suggested that we use a water bottle to squirt him when he acted out. We faithfully tried each intervention. Mark took the lead with Jasper on our outings since Jasper's flailing required a degree of strength to even get the leash under one's foot during an episode. I was grateful for his role, since I found the looks of disapproval and fear from onlookers during these public displays too difficult to manage. During many training outings to PetSmart, Jasper could be heard throughout the store as he screamed at the top of his lungs while Mark dutifully stood on his leash, patiently waiting for the temper tantrum to end. During walks it was common for Jasper to be completely drenched from the water bottle, water dripping comically from the tips of his ears, as he continued to wail and flop around as Mark did his best to shorten his leash by stepping on it. We tried treats and blocking his view from what triggered the outburst. Jasper only became more irritated and continued his high pitched scream as he desperately ducked and weaved to see the desired object. While Mark and I laughed about the episodes in private, it was a difficult time. Mark had taken over this part of Jasper's training and was beginning to admit the toll the public humiliation was taking. Jasper continued his Jekyll and Hyde persona; he was a model student in a controlled classroom setting, but he displayed uncontrolled antics in everyday public places.

At times I wondered if I would have to give up my dreams of working with Jasper as a therapy dog. How could this out-of-control dog ever overcome this? Despite our frequent tales of failure, Ashley never seemed overly concerned. She patiently encouraged us to keep going. With time, Mark was able to help Jasper manage his behavior on occasion. During our walks each week, there were times when Jasper could calmly walk by another dog or even a skater. On rarer occasions, we were able to sit and watch a dog and person play Frisbee or a dog run after a ball from a distance. These were always near the end of our walks, but still, amazing progress given our history! Encouraged by Mark's success, I resumed some of the public training. With time, I was able to walk with Jasper without major incident. We still had the occasional outburst, but they were readily correctable. Jasper (and, more importantly, I) seemed to be getting the hang of it. Mark often challenged me to push Jasper further, walking closer to a potential trigger. However, though I was relieved at the progress we had made I was still fearful of losing control, so I usually shied away.

On a September day one full year from when we first met

our little Jasper, he passed the Delta Society Pet Partner test. He wasn't perfect. He had the occasional outburst when he first saw the dog who would play the part of the "neutral dog" in the test or when he saw the stuffed "dancing chicken" he would have to ignore as part of this test, but he got it together. His love of people and his joy in being a part of a group of humans were clearly evident. I could not have been prouder of the little dude. Since then he has joined his brother Rocky as a therapy dog at the local health department, working one full day each week. Staff and clients frequently note how different his personality is from his stoic brother. He is more demonstrative in his enthusiasm as he wags his entire back end during a visit or catches his ball on command. He is always ready to visit or show off his tricks, always ready with an endearing doggy smile. Many even pick Jasper as their favorite for his playful personality and reputation for making an occasional mistake. They enjoy seeing his "human" side. However, because of his high herding and prey drive, I am always on alert to ensure that he is successful and nothing triggers an outburst. Sudden movements are still far too fun to Jasper, and risk triggering his instincts. He is rated as "predictable," which means that he needs his environment to remain calm, and it is my role as his handler to manage his environment to help him succeed.

Just this last year, it was time for Jasper to be re-evaluated (Delta Society therapy animal teams are re-evaluated every two years to ensure they remain safe and appropriate visitors). With two full years of working under our belt, I was confident this test would be a piece of cake. Then, to my surprise, Jasper struggled with several elements of the test. He was not as focused and at times was not as confident as he had been two years ago. While he passed the test, it was a difficult realization for me. I had become complacent in my training with Jasper; I had allowed him to become "good enough." I realized that I had stopped pushing him, and had found a way to work only within our comfort zone.

While this was wise in a work setting, it was not helpful in assisting him to continue to learn to manage the unexpected in life. When pushed passed this zone (as in the test), Jasper lacked confidence and began to exhibit some old behaviors. I had let him down.

After much soul searching, I signed Jasper up for agility classes. I knew this would be a challenge. The primary situations in which Jasper continues to struggle are those in which there are children or dogs running in close proximity to him. Agility would place us in the heart of such a situation. While I playfully asked the instructor before signing up for the class if they would be able to handle it if Jasper screamed and threw himself on the floor during the class, I was ill prepared for what truly happened.

It was a cold, snowy Colorado day when Jasper and I arrived at our first agility class. The facility is known for training AKC champions, and the trainers made it clear from the beginning that they were going to ensure that participants knew how to execute each obstacle according to the AKC rule book. Out of nervousness, I quietly joked to Jasper that he didn't have to do it so perfectly. We were there to just have fun, not to learn to compete. Jasper dutifully looked up at me in response then resumed visiting with the other dogs near by. He was excited by the surroundings, but remained in complete control. It was a dream compared to the nightmare of the little pup I had adopted three years earlier. He was a model citizen, politely visiting and responding obediently when I asked him to lie down and ignore his new classmates. And then the class began.

Within the first fifteen minutes of class, the chaos level rose to a point that Jasper could no longer handle. Much to my horror, he began to lunge and growl when another dog ran past. I quickly struggled to control him, embarrassed by his outbursts. I was sure he was not being aggressive, but it was hard to convince strangers of this. I muttered apologies and tried to explain to anyone who was within ear shot that we were here due to this

very problem. "Jasper's a good dog. He just gets overstimulated."
Unfazed by my explanations, other owners pulled their dogs away
from Jasper and gave me that look that implies, "Control your
dog!" At one point, sensing other participants' apprehension, one
of the instructors stopped the class and, to my relief, announced,
"Jasper is not a mean dog. He just has a very high prey drive."
Jasper flawlessly completed each agility task, only to lunge and
bark despite my best efforts as the other dogs went by while he
waited his turn to do his task again. The break could not have
come soon enough. I could no longer hold back my tears. It was
humiliating. "He's a well trained dog! I tried to explain to the
instructor between my tears. We just have this one issue ..." The
more I tried to explain the more the tears flowed. All the while
Jasper looked up with concern wondering what could possibly be
making me so upset.

The trainer, in a kind but firm voice, said, "No one is yelling
at you. He is fine. You need to leave your emotions in the car."
We got through the rest of the class. It wasn't pretty, but we did
it. The following week I was much more prepared for what was
in store. I was also determined that, no matter what, I had to
keep it together. My feelings of embarrassment and humiliation
were only making matters worse. It was time to work through
this. Jasper deserved for us both to learn to manage the tough
emotions and situations. Avoiding them only got us so far. It was
time to move past them.

By the third class, I was starting to see improvements. I was
able to redirect Jasper when he got overstimulated, and he was
able to keep his focus on me when other dogs went running past.
Huge steps, but more were ahead. The next tasks required that
the dogs work off leash. I did my best to just remove Jasper's leash
for his turn, only to return it promptly when he was finished.
I was terrified to lose control and having him running around
the room terrorizing everyone. It was during one of these times
that I was holding things up, fumbling with the leash, that the

instructor hollered, "Lose the leash! Do you think you really need it?" She added an eye roll for effect. Stunned, I started to mumble that yes indeed I did think I needed it, when I thought better of that response. I tossed the leash toward the wall, took a deep breath, and worked to control Jasper with just a tab (a short leash used to grab the dog if needed when working off leash). True to my fears, he did run off a little later. Jasper escaped to run up the A-frame and through the tire jump, but then he quickly returned when I called. I was shocked—not that he ran off, but that he returned when called even with so many other dogs around. The following week he escaped yet again when our group was working on jumps and the other group was working on the A-frame and tunnel (his favorite). Much to my embarrassment, he jumped over the retaining wall to join the other group, but when I called him, he jumped back over the same retaining wall (only after joyfully running over the A-frame and saying hello to a classmate) to obediently return with a big doggy smile on his face.

Jasper and I are far from resolving these issues. He still barks and lunges when his prey drive is triggered, and I am still embarrassed when people respond with fear and judgment. At the time of this writing, we are still actively involved in various types of training classes and are working each week to better manage our emotions in these areas. We are making progress. Jasper has been my little gift from heaven. He is the gift I never would have been willing to accept had I known what was in store. Yet how grateful I am for him and the lessons he has brought. He has forced me to learn to grow in public, no matter how embarrassing the situation might be. He is teaching me that there is so much in life we miss out on when we are only willing to learn and try new things in safe, private settings. With the humiliation comes pride at a job well done. Jasper is an expert at being himself and not worrying about what people think. I would be wise to learn from him. He is teaching me that one can only grow so much while remaining safe. The rest requires risk. It is impossible to be Jasper's partner and not be indelibly changed. For that, I am forever grateful.

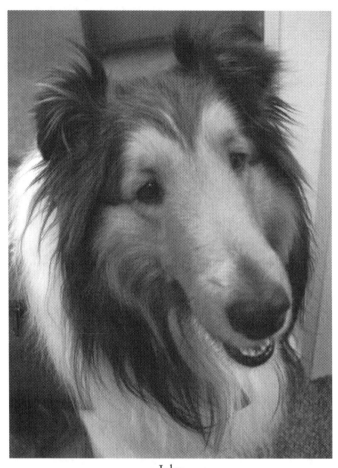

Jake
*Photo by Mark Hochstedler*

# Chapter Seven
# Jake and Willie

*One reason a dog can be such
a comfort when you're feeling
blue is that he doesn't try to
find out why.*

— Anonymous

As I began the incredible journey of writing this book, I had some vague notions of the types of stories I was looking for, but the details remained unclear, and I knew defining what I wanted would be a process all in itself. All I knew for sure was that I deeply believed that each and every therapy dog handler had been profoundly changed through this process of working with a canine partner, and that each continued this work for a very personal reason. I didn't know what each person's reason was, but I believed there was one. I hoped to discover these reasons, and to then transform them into heartwarming stories that would in turn transform the reader. One of the first people who offered his story was Rich. I eagerly braved the cold Colorado weather to drive well over an hour to the medical center where he and his two shelties volunteer. He was easy to spot as I entered the building. He was smiling and chatting away with the information desk worker, as his dog, Jake, seemed content to watch those passing by. After brief introductions, we retreated into the volunteers' office, and before I could even open my pad of paper or grab my pen, Rich started sharing all the wonderful experiences and thoughts about working with his two therapy dogs. His was a story that was eagerly and proudly told.

I found myself desperate to slow him down so I would not miss an important thought or fact. I frantically wrote each word

I could, but knew there was no way I could capture all that he spoke. He jumped from story to story, and told each with colorful descriptions, all the while wearing a wide smile. He seemed to pause and look to me on occasion for effect, and then just as quickly continued on with more stories. At times, I tried to steer Rich gently toward the topic of my book, curious to learn just what difference working with these two dogs had made for him personally. Each time, he paused as though I was interrupting what was truly important, but he didn't answer my questions. On one occasion, he simply said, "Dogs don't ask me the questions you do. That's why I do this." I was puzzled by his answer and didn't really comprehend how it connected to my question, but I decided to just keep listening. Clearly there was a story here, and I hoped in time I would hear it. I soon determined it was best simply to listen, for here was a man who was clearly passionate about his work. There was something so engaging about his passion. Jake seemed oblivious to the conversation. He lay on the floor, and seemed content to just be. He was adorable. I found myself wanting to sit on the floor with him and enjoy him, but I knew I needed to stay focused and gather my facts in order to capture the story Rich was offering.

I learned that Rich had always had dogs. However, like so many (including me) he did not really understand nor appreciate the power that dogs held until much later in life. As he described it, he didn't understand their "dogness" when he was a child. He didn't understand them as a different species or understand the importance of truly caring for them through proper grooming, walks, training, etc. I could tell that something had changed as he became older, but I just couldn't figure it out. Sure, there was a maturing in his relationships with dogs that is necessary for anyone to partner with a working dog in a professional setting, but why? Why the shift? It eluded me. So I kept listening.

He told me about his "forever dog," Tyler, who broke Rich's heart when he died on his daughter's birthday, a date he will always remember for reasons both happy and sad. He soon decided to adopt a dog to help with his grief, and he contacted the Colorado Sheltie Rescue. He knew that younger dogs had much better odds of finding a good home, so he decided to adopt an older dog as a thank you to Tyler. So, on his own birthday the family made arrangements for a potential dog to be brought to their home. Even before meeting the dog, Rich and his wife had already decided they would agree to the adoption as long as the dog was mobile in any way. When Jenni arrived from the rescue, she brought eleven-and-a-half-year-old Willie. No sooner had they given their consent for the adoption, a second sheltie snuck through the door. It was two-year-old Jake, who was traveling with Jenni and was moving from one foster home to another. Jake had experienced a difficult life. He was emaciated, had a vacant look in his eyes, and fur that was in desperate need of attention. Jake had been on the lam before he ended up at the shelter, and he was not accustomed to being around people. His previous owners had had little to no contact with him, and had received multiple citations for "dog at large." Jake finally received some much needed attention when the neighbors overheard Jake's owners discussing drowning little Jake so that they would not have to pay the accumulating fines. It was a heartrending story, which immediately tugged at Rich's heart strings. Two dogs weren't in the plan, but Rich instantly knew he wanted them both. At once, he turned to his wife and started to plead his case. He promised to be the one to train them both (she had always done all the dog training), and insisted that this would be the best birthday present ever if he could just have them both. She gave in and the pair became his. As he told me this story, he said he later regretted making that statement to his wife, since he now realized that it somehow implied that the previous birthday presents were not as great as what he picked out for himself.

At last I interrupted Rich to explore how he ended up doing therapy dog work, and he politely stopped and then refocused his storytelling as I requested. He always gets into things backward, he explained. His wife, Karyn, has the rare disease lymphangio-leiomyomatosis (LAM), which is a progressive and frequently fatal lung disease, and she travels regularly to the National Institute of Health in Maryland for treatment. Although living with a chronic and possibly fatal disease seemed significant to me, Rich said this just as a matter of fact and continued on with the story. He did later hand me a brochure about LAM and made it clear that he is very proud of his wife for working to bring more public recognition to the disease. During one of her treatments, she was visited by a therapy dog, and she was impressed enough by the experience to share it with Rich. She even brought home a Polaroid of the therapy dog to show him. Soon after, Rich met a volunteer handler and therapy dog at the local senior fair while he was getting a flu shot. They struck up a conversation, and Rich decided to learn more about therapy dog work. He took his golden retriever, Bo, and his new pup Willie, and took his first stab at the therapy dog exam. It was a humbling experience, and after failing his first try, he decided to work privately with a service dog trainer to learn how to better partner with his canine buddies. During this process he discovered that Bo was too stressed in such settings, so he decided to focus his attention on Jake and Willie. As Rich so eloquently states, "I learned that I had to be trained. I had to learn to be a handler." Rich stuck with it, and it paid off. They passed.

Rich told me about countless visits with his patients in the senior center Alzheimer's unit. There were patients who were not talking much before their visit but would suddenly make efforts to communicate when they saw the dog, and others who were eager to introduce their new canine friend to others on the unit. Rich explained how these patients would frequently tell him all about their own dogs of days gone by, only to forget they had just told the story and start telling it from the beginning once again. Rich smiled as he said that he would pretend he'd never heard the story before since the stories allowed the patients to be themselves once again. It is all they have left as the merciless Alzheimer's robs them of their current memories. Rich told me how he works with patients who are quiet; how he waits them out, trusting that they would respond. "They always do," he told me. During these visits he sees heart rates begin to rest as he observes the sophisticated machines that measure the patients' heart rate and oxygen levels. These machines provide objective testament to the difference that he feels in his own heart that he and his dogs are making for others. He told other moving stories such as the one when he was visiting a patient who was in a coma in the Intensive Care Unit. He was invited to visit the patient, and he put the patient's hand on the dog. The patient then moved for the first time in three weeks. There was the ninety-eight-year-old woman who was so excited to visit with Jake, she kept saying, "I love you Jake!" Jake, who does not lick when working, broke his own rule and gave the kind woman a big kiss before leaving for the day. As Rich and Jake left the woman's room, the nurse comforted the woman by saying, "It's time to go to sleep and dream about Jake." Stories such as these leave Rich with what he calls *kvell,* a Jewish word meaning to beam with pride and pleasure.

In between these wonderful stories, I gently pushed to learn how working with Jake and Willie has changed Rich. He again seemed slightly irritated that I would divert our time away from his cherished dogs to focus on him. On one such occasion he told me that he enjoyed working with the dogs because he was able to be anonymous. "The patients don't ask about me," he said, "they just focus on the dogs." He then went on to tell me about a wonderful woman he and Jake had visited, who was a Delta Society Pet Partner in Sacramento. She had spotted Rich and Jake across the room, and had quickly approached to inquire if they would accompany her to the fourth floor to visit her sister. How could he say no? As they made their way to her sister's room, the woman explained that her sister was gravely ill and only had a few weeks or months left to live. Rich set Jake up on the bed to visit. The following day, Rich and Willie went again to visit the sister, but were instead greeted by the woman herself. She told Rich that her sister had suddenly passed away only a half hour before. She gave Willie a big hug and cried. They stayed and visited for quite some time. The woman said that the circle was now complete. She had been visiting all these years with her own dog, giving comfort to those in need. Now in need of comfort herself, she could personally experience the joy that comes from a visit from a therapy dog.

As our time was drawing to an end, I tried one more time to learn the difference that working with these dogs had made to Rich. He then told me about the love the two dogs have for each other. He told the story of one morning when Jake came and woke him up at 5:00 a.m. to let him know that Willie was unable to get up the back stairs and through the doggie door. Willie needed help, and Jake made sure Rich knew it. It was then that he commented that he cries around his dogs and they lick his tears away. He quickly added, "I don't cry much." He told me that maybe working with his dogs is a midlife crisis, one in which he is doing good for others. And with that, our time together was over. I enjoyed the interview, but left with more questions than answers. I was no closer to understanding how working with these dogs had truly changed Rich. At one point in our conversation Rich told me that he did stand-up comedy as a hobby. In this role, his job was to make people laugh and to use what they said to one-up them by using it in his act. I could really see how Rich would be great at that. There was something about him that was wonderful to hear—engaging stories, yet personally distant. Talking to Rich that day was like watching pebbles skip across a beautiful lake. There is a magic and beauty to the skipping and the resultant ripples, but the process does not allow one to understand or discover what lies under the water. How could I use his story without this crucial element? I knew that during this journey I would be told stories that I would later decide I could not use. That is part of the process. Yet for some reason, there seemed to be something to Rich's story that kept me from just letting it go.

I continued to struggle with what to do with Rich's story for the next couple of months. I received an occasional e-mail from Rich telling me of touching encounters that he and his pups had during visits. After much thought, I finally decided that I might as well question him just a little further. Something was keeping him connected and wanting to share his story. "What's the worst that could happen? If he doesn't respond to my e-mail, then I'm no worse for the wear," I decided. And so I carefully crafted an e-mail asking the tough questions. I asked about his wife's disease. When was she diagnosed? What was it like? How did it change things for them both? What difference did the dogs make for Karyn and Rich during this process? These were just a few of the questions I asked. So many questions. They were the kind of questions that my mother would have been embarrassed for me to ask, embarrassed that I would pry into such personal matters. However, it needed to be done, I told myself; it was my journalistic duty. I hit the send button, and then waited. Rich quickly responded and told me that he was happy to answer and that he and Karyn would find a time to discuss them and get back with me. I waited … and waited. Just when I had decided that I had probably pushed too far, the e-mail came.

It was an e-mail that touched my soul, for there … was Rich's heart. He told me of the first signs of Karyn's disease, how her lung collapsed first in 1980 and then again in 1981. How at the very time that they finally conceived their first child after trying so very long, they learned that her lung had collapsed once again and x-rays were needed despite the pregnancy. Just at the time that the couple should have been able to enjoy the birth of their child, they had to face the effects of continued health problems and the unknown. He told me how scary and painful it was during the seven years before they learned what was causing her breathing difficulties, and about how devastating and sad the actual diagnosis was. He spoke about how LAM has changed their lives in every way. Karyn is currently waiting for a double lung transplant, and Rich has moved into the role of helper and supporter in all areas of life. I could tell from the e-mail how much he deeply loves his wife and how he gladly would do anything to help. He described in his colorful way having to learn to do all the chores that he previously left for his wife, and having to juggle earning a living, keeping up the house, and being emotionally present for her. He wrote, "I try not to get lectured about ruining any of Karyn's delicates," and in the next sentence he wrote, "I love her so, and it hurts. It hurts to see your forever love struggling."

Here I found the answers to my questions about how he is different because of his dogs. In this e-mail, he wrote about how much he hates to think and talk about the pain and the impending loss of his beloved Karyn. He writes,

> I know I have channeled my emotions to the dogs. It is my way of detaching. We do fight about this, Karyn saying, I'm not dead, I'm here. Dogs don't need emotions, dogs do not talk. I do not need to be conversational with my dogs. My dogs just care that I am present. I know I do not discuss with Karyn her disease most times. Unless asked. I avoid it. I avoid anything emotional. Clean the house. Take out the trash. Pick up the poop. Avoidance.

At this moment I realized that Rich had been answering my question all along. As a psychotherapist by trade, I am usually very good at hearing what is in a person's heart. That is one of my gifts. As I train other therapists, I frequently remind them that if they miss what a person is saying that is most important to them, they should simply keep listening. The person will keep repeating it until they finally hear it. As I looked back on my notes from my time with Rich, I now saw the answer scattered throughout my writing. He was repeating it over and over until I heard it. "My dogs don't ask me these questions." "I'm able to be anonymous. They don't ask me questions. They just enjoy the dogs." There was my answer. The dogs provide an outlet for Rich to connect with people in a very meaningful way while providing the protection of his heart that he desperately needs. What a gift those dogs give to Rich on a daily basis! They give Rich the strength to face each day. They give him an outlet for his pain, while simultaneously accepting his need to keep his emotions private.

I also learned through Rich's e-mail he wants to learn to be more emotionally present for his wife. He went on to say that because of his circumstances he is more aware of and responsive to the needs of others. "Pet therapy blurs the line between giving and receiving—this is my gift and pet therapy restoreth my soul." Rich's story is now one of my favorites, for it proves true my belief that it is the handler who receives the greatest gift when working with a therapy dog. Although it is always easy to see the difference that a therapy dog makes to those they visit, it is only by delving just a little deeper that we uncover incredible stories of how the love of a dog truly transforms and heals our souls.

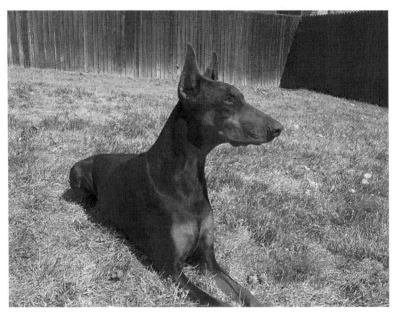

Bogey
*Photo by Shannon Johnson*

# Chapter Eight
# Bogie

*Dogs find our soft spots,*
*keeping us in touch with a more*
*honest vision of ourselves that*
*doesn't buy its own façade.*

*—Monks of New Skete*

Why is it that as humans we judge others by how they look? We all know that this is not fair or even right, but still, on some level we all are guilty of these superficial impressions. When I first got my sable and white rough coat collie, Rocky, everyone immediately fell in love with him. He was charismatic even at three months old, and had a movie-star quality that continues to this day. It was commonplace for strangers to approach and spontaneously begin to share some childhood memory about collies. They seemed to be drawn to his adorable puppy face and his perfect markings. He was amazingly photogenic, and even the most candid pictures seemed professionally staged (which was advantageous for us since we are camera challenged). Now that he has matured into an adult dog and become a Lassie-lookalike, he continues to draw attention, and comments about his outward beauty are commonplace.

When our second dog, Jasper, joined our family, I was struck by the difference in people's reactions. Although the collie rescue insisted that he is a rough coat collie, we have determined that he is most likely a rough coat mix (most likely with a border collie or an Aussie). He never had the characteristic look of a thorough-bred rough coat collie, and although he was four months old when we brought him home, he just wasn't as attention-stopping cute as most puppies are. In addition, Jasper was cursed with a right ear that constantly flopped over his head like a bad comb-over. His foster mother at the rescue had used fabric glue in a feeble attempt to coax it into a tulip-tipped shape, but somehow it only made it look more ridiculous and added a glob of hard fur-incrusted substance at the tip of his ear as it lay on the top of his head like a hat. His coat was dull and coarse, far from the expected fuzzy soft fur one would have expected in his breed. He simply looked like a small adult dog with a malformed ear, and strangers treated him as such, hardly giving him a second glance. Only his razor sharp baby teeth and his playful spirit gave testimony to his true age.

I will never forget the look that one of my co-workers gave me when I brought my new puppy to meet them and introduce him as a possible future therapy dog. Before this meeting, I had only described him as the cute four-month-old rough coat collie puppy I had adopted. After being exposed to Rocky's baby pictures, it was clear that this co-worker had a preconceived idea of what Jasper would look like as she shot me one of those surprised, I-better-not-say-something-otherwise-I-will-hurt-your-feelings looks. She cautiously asked, "What is on his ear?" and then pulled her hand away in a poorly disguised act of disgust. Nonetheless, I saw something in that awkward, gangly puppy that would not be dissuaded.

We were eventually able to tame Jasper's wayward ear, and his coat now has the lustrous shine of good health and proper grooming, but Jasper will never be kind to the camera lens; he still looks like he is being beaten in most of his photographs. However, he has matured into a fine young therapy dog who embodies the curiosity and thirst for people that are the hallmarks of the job. Although Jasper was not what most people first envisioned, he continues to have talents and traits that far surpass his outwardly perfect brother, Rocky. First impressions can be deceiving.

In devising the concept for this book, I was not sure whom I would meet or what stories I would hear throughout the process.

It was an adventure. One such chapter in this adventure began with a simple e-mail, short and to the point. A woman named Shannon stated that she trained and worked with a therapy/service dog and would be willing to tell her story if I was interested. I was struck by the lack of information that this e-mail contained. It was all the info I truly needed, but it was remarkably short by comparison to the others I had received. I had come to learn that therapy dog handlers frequently are very excited about their dogs and the work they do together and often give lots of information about the dog's breed, work, name, etc., without any prompting on my part. I was also confused by the description of "therapy/service dog." These are very different types of working dogs, and I was unsure what to make of this dual description. I arranged a time to meet Shannon, still not sure if she was truly the handler for the dog, or simply an employee at the agency that worked alongside the canine. Either way, I could not pass up the offer for a good story.

As I pulled up to the residential child treatment center, I was struck by the stateliness of the building. It was a beautiful mansion-looking brick building built upon a hill and overlooking the rest of the residential neighborhood. As I walked up the stairs and opened the heavy iron security door, I could not help but feel highly visible. This was not a place one could quietly sneak into. Although I had been familiar with this residential facility and the quality work they do in the Denver area for my entire twenty-year career, I had never actually seen the facility. Everything about it was shattering my preconceived notions. As I sat in the old fashioned sitting room waiting to meet Shannon and her canine buddy, I was struck by how incongruent the setting felt with the population the agency serves. The building and furnishings were from many years ago, and had been preserved in a way that gave them a museum-like quality, eloquence, and formality. It reminded me of a grandmother's parlor. The floor boards creaked with age as staff members walked through the halls, giving the building character that only comes with age. By contrast, this agency provides services to the youth of our community who have nowhere else to turn. The building houses up to twenty-seven troubled ten- to eighteen-year-old male clients. Many are gang members whose paths have crossed societal or legal limits; others are victims who have gone on to become perpetrators of untold forms of abuse. All have painful stories to tell, and all need the professional guidance of the staff of this facility to help them get their lives back on track. Working in a setting such as this is a thankless job, for the clients are in need of the most intensive forms of treatment, and frequently require physical restraints and limits to change their ways of behaving and interacting with the world.

My thoughts were interrupted by loud steps approaching, accompanied by the clatter of nails on the wood floor. It is an unmistakable sound to a dog lover such as me. I don't know exactly what I was expecting, but what I saw was definitely not it. As I turned to look I was greeted by an intimidating eighty-pound red Doberman pinscher wearing a vest clearly labeled "Service Dog," with his handler, Shannon, in tow. The dog's enthusiasm and power were unmistakable, as Shannon, while clearly still in full control of the dog, was moving in partnership with the sheer mass of the dog. Bogie was very friendly, and acted just like any other therapy dog I have ever met; friendly, sweet, and eager to interact. He gave me a wonderful doggie smile as I petted his head and let him sniff my hand. How could anyone not love this dog? During this initial introduction, I found myself asking myself, "What was I really expecting, a poodle? Maybe a Pomeranian? Why was I not expecting such a magnificent animal?" It was a rude reminder that I, too—unbeknownst to me—have preconceived ideas about therapy dogs and people. Shannon, true to her no-nonsense e-mails, said simply, "Hello. This is Bogie," and ushered me into a conference room. She took a chair calmly and confidently and silently waited for me to begin. Bogie was less than subtle as he pushed his weight against my leg and rested his heavy head in my lap, clearly wanting me to pet him and give him lots of attention. What a pussy cat. And so Shannon began to tell me their story.

Shannon had put a significant amount of thought into what kind of dog she wanted to get. She had hopes of someday training her dog to be a therapy dog once he settled down, but she really just wanted a family pet for her and her husband, a dog who would also guard the house in their absence. She considered the standard contenders (Labrador retriever, golden retriever, German shepherd), but then decided that those breeds had far too much hair and would be too troublesome to maintain in a work setting. So she began to look into getting a Doberman. She had initially hoped to get a black female since she had heard that females were better with children. After completing some research, she spoke with a breeder who had one puppy left. It was a red male, but he had been specially temperament tested and previously selected to be a service dog for a gentleman in Salt Lake City. At the last minute the man had changed his mind in favor of a black puppy. Although the color and sex were not Shannon's ideal, she was quick to understand that the puppy's temperament was key to her ambitions (she had also learned that males can be equally good with kids). The puppy became hers, and they have not looked back.

A co-worker encouraged Shannon to look into psychiatric service dog training to work with some clients at another agency at which also Shannon worked. And so the idea was born, and Shannon began the time-consuming task of training a service dog. Even though Shannon had never trained a dog before, she was up for the challenge. She took some basic obedience classes with Bogie, bought a couple of books, and then struck out on her own to learn the skills a well-trained service dog required. She and Bogie went everywhere together—the movies, museums, grocery shopping, the Vegas strip, Epcot, airplane trips, etc. It was a daunting job. Somewhere along the line came the idea to bring Bogie to work at the residential treatment program.

Shannon's agency had ventured into the world of animal-assisted therapy once before. It was in the 1990s, prior to Shannon's employment there. They had a Labrador retriever who resided at the residential facility in an effort to add some normalcy to the environment for the adolescent boys. Unfortunately, the fate of the lab was similar to that of many dogs placed into this kind of setting, even with the best of intentions. Staff who were already overworked and underpaid had little time to provide the necessary care to another creature, and the dog became neglected. Even worse, the dog fell victim to many of the residents who had a history of cruelty to animals. As Shannon described him, "He was everyone's victim." The administration wisely decided that having a dog present in the facility was not fair to the dog, and not something they wanted to revisit. However, when Shannon began working at the facility she understood the power of the human-animal bond, and looked for ways in which the boys and staff could benefit from a therapy dog, while protecting the animal. She soon discovered that confidentiality issues meant they couldn't even bring in volunteer animal-handler teams. She then considered the possibility of using her own dog as a psychiatric service dog. This would allow the dog to accompany her and her clients on the many recreational outings that are a routine part of her day as a recreational therapist. It would also provide the protection that the dog needed, since it would be her family pet, going home with her each evening.

Bogie's breed as a Doberman only helped as this plan developed, for as Shannon explained, smiling, "When you think about abusing a dog, you don't think about abusing a Doberman." It was also this tough exterior that helped endear Bogie to the clients. Since many of the kids were gang members, they pride themselves on being tough, the kind of person that no one wants to mess with. Bogie fit this tough-guy image. He looked like a tough-guy gangster, and was someone the kids could respect for that very reason. They could see themselves in him. Yet, just like the boys themselves, Bogie was a softy deep inside. This meant the boys protected him, ensuring that Bogie is well treated. "The worst thing they do is feed him under the table (which in their minds is good for him)," says Shannon. The only harm that has come his way is when one of the boys forgets to look where he is walking or moving a chair and bumps or steps on Bogie. The other kids are then quick to chastise the inconsiderate boy, and remind him to watch out for their pal. The boys act better when Bogie is around, almost seeming to set a good example for their canine friend.

As a service dog, Bogie was specially trained to perform various tasks. One of the tasks Shannon taught Bogie was how to open an unlocked door. Now, most dog lovers would never dream of teaching their dogs such a task, but it was the perfect job for Bogie. The residential facility is a locked facility, meaning that clients are not allowed to leave without permission, and staff have the authority to use physical force, if need be, to restrain the clients to prevent them from harming themselves or others. This can present many difficulties for staff when chaos erupts, for it can take all available staff members to physically manage the clients. In a crisis, this can leave no one available to unlock the door to allow necessary assistance (such as from the police) into the facility. Bogie was just the answer to this problem. If Bogie could unlock a door and allow someone to enter upon command, he could free the staff members to attend to the unruly boys.

While lockdowns are relatively rare occurrences, Bogie has a very important role on a daily basis, for his very presence has a calming effect on the boys. According to Shannon, Bogie seems to know which of the boys have the most severe mental illness, and he prefers to be with them. While one would think that Bogie would like to be with the calmer, more loving and manageable boys, that is not the case. He seems to know who needs him the most and seeks to be with those individuals. When one of the boys becomes upset, the boy will begin to dissociate and become detached from reality. Bogie then pushes his body into the boy to encourage him to pet him. This very act of petting Bogie has a calming effect and brings the boy back into reality. This interaction results in the client's voice and breathing slowing and returning to normal.

During one such incident, Shannon was in a restaurant with her clients and Bogie when two of her boys became engaged in an altercation with two girls. Bogie moved into action from his usual position under the table, standing up and placing his head on the knee of one of the boys who was most escalated. Before that day, this boy had had no use for Bogie. He considered himself to be "too cool" to interact with the dog; however, at this moment he looked down at Bogie and began to pet his head. By doing so, the boy was able to calm himself down, continuing to pet Bogie while the other kid continued to escalate.

When they are on a therapeutic outing, the kids from the facility are rarely a welcome sight within the community. They are dressed in gang colors and are frequently judged by those around them as unruly and potential trouble. Before Bogie's arrival, the only interaction these kids often had with those in the community was reprimands and negative looks. These negative interactions only served to heighten the distance the kids felt from mainstream society. Bogie has had a positive impact on this now that he accompanies the boys on most outings. Thanks to Bogie, the boys are frequently approached by others, curious about the role of the dog. This gives the boys many more opportunities to practice their social skills by introducing the dog or explaining his role. Through interactions such as these, the boys gain confidence in their skills and are able to walk away with a positive experience.

One of these interactions occurred when Shannon took one of the boys to register as a sex offender as Colorado law requires.

Now, one has to realize that these boys have not had many positive interactions with the police or the legal system. They have been on the wrong side of the law, and have experienced firsthand the harshness and disdain that comes from violating societal limits. Likewise, the police officers have often formed a negative opinion about boys who dress and act like the clients of the facility, for they have been the ones responsible for protecting the innocent from boys such as these. While the young man and Shannon were waiting, a police officer approached them to ask about Bogie. Soon several law enforcement officers were gathered with them, all talking about dogs. In any other setting, the boy would have been extremely uncomfortable, and the police officers most likely would not have initiated this pleasant conversation. However, due to Bogie's presence, the boy and the law enforcement officers were able to have a seemingly normal conversation about the joy of having a dog—something this child sorely needed in order to change how he perceives law enforcement as he works toward becoming a contributing member of society in the future.

Dogs have a way of drawing the attention of others to themselves, thereby pulling the attention away from people and things that otherwise would have been the focus of question or judgment. It is this trait that allows the residential clients to enter into community settings without the previous suspicions or to comfortably join previously unwelcome conversations. When I questioned Shannon about how working with Bogie has changed her as an individual, it was this very quality to which she referred. She spoke about her husband, who is six foot eleven inches tall. She said curious children frequently comment on his height, despite their parents' embarrassment. But there is a marked difference when Bogie is in tow, for the children's attention (and therefore their impromptu comments) is on the dog saying, "Hey, look at that dog!" It is hard to blend in when Bogie is present, Shannon says. Because of Bogie, Shannon is well known by those throughout the large organization as the "lady with the dog." Bogie brings everyone around him out of isolation, and yet simultaneously takes uncomfortable focus away from the individual.

As I talked with Shannon, I noticed that she couldn't really put into words how Bogie has changed her, but she knew she had indeed been changed. Many people with whom I have spoken throughout the journey of this book have been taken aback by my question about how working with their therapy dog has changed them. They want to tell me all about the dog, believing that this is the true story. When I push them further they seem confused and say they really are no different, and then refocus onto the dog. This was not the case with Shannon. Each time I pushed her on the subject, she became more thoughtful and gave me a few more nuggets about how she is different because of Bogie—more patient, more attentive of her clients, more outgoing, more aware of the power of service dogs. She even told me of her dreams to train additional service dogs now that she has discovered she has this previously unrecognized ability.

As I wrapped up my visit with Shannon and Bogie I was struck by the reminder never to judge a book by its cover, for one never knows the wonderful treasures that lie within. While Bogie looks so tough and intimidating on the surface, that's not who he really is and what is in his heart—just like the boys he watches over each day. Likewise, Shannon's demeanor, initially so pragmatic and matter-of-fact, now gave way to a softer side as she explained, "It's like he's working miracles each day, and I'm seeing it." Their pragmatic exterior is so perfect for their clientele, it is only when one gets closer that the genuine compassion they bring shines through the tough-guy façade. They are a consummate team, offering a timely reminder to look beyond the surface and into the hearts of those we meet.

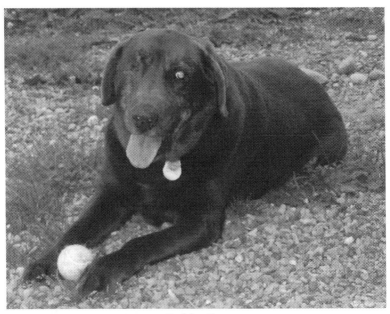

Bobby Lee
*Photo by Peggy Menze*

# Chapter Nine
# Bobby Lee

*One reason a dog is such a
lovable creature is his tail wags
instead of his tongue.*

—Anonymous

As humans, our ability to understand, reason, and intellectualize is very important. It is because of these traits that we are able to create, develop, reason, and solve problems. Unfortunately, these same characteristics that are the foundation of what makes us human also make us vulnerable for thinking ourselves into a funk when bad things happen. Because we understand how others may perceive us, or that possible opportunities might be limited due to our current resources or life circumstance, we are at increased risk to awfulize. Humans are prone to worry about how we compare to others, to do the "what ifs," and the "what could have beens." How easy it is to become depressed or discouraged when the unexpected happen or when challenges come our way. It is tempting at times to even entertain the unhelpful question, "Why me?" So is it any real surprise to hear that the people who are most successful in this world have somehow learned how to take life as it comes? They hope for the best, but prepare for the worst. They have somehow learned to prevent what is preventable, and then accept what comes their way. As the old saying goes, they have learned to make lemonade out of lemons. It is the art of living a happy life. Unfortunately, not all humans have developed this skill.

Animals do not have the same reasoning powers as humans, and this actually protects them. They have an incredible gift of just being. When problems come, the problem just is. Nothing

113

more. They don't question what they did to deserve such a fate, or seek to determine blame. They simply find the best way to cope with the challenge at hand. This trait is at the heart of their incredible ability to forgive and give unconditional love to those around them. They have an uncanny ability to keep life simple and in perspective. Because of these basic facts about humans and animals, I was eager to speak with Peggy when she contacted me about her very special therapy dog, Bobby Lee. Here is his story.

Although Peggy had never had a dog as a child, she and her first husband did have a golden retriever, and then later a cocker spaniel. But life with three kids can be hectic, and although the dogs were present, they took a back seat to the hustle and bustle that consumed their lives. Peggy really didn't have the time for the dogs, and the dogs were simply there. As time passed, the children became older, and life was changed by divorce. Living happily in Chicago, Peggy met her new husband. Soon after they married they decided it was time to get a dog. Her husband had grown up with a yellow lab and their neighbors at that time also had a lab, so they had become fond of the breed. They researched available rescues and found a wonderful black lab, whom they named Alex. During this process Peggy became friends with the rescue worker, so when it was time a year later to further expand their family, Peggy knew who to call. Her friend told her about a wonderful chocolate lab who needed a good home.

The lab had had a really rough start in life. He had been found wandering around in the Ozark Mountains of Arkansas by a kind woman. She was walking up her drive one evening when she saw a large, dark beast nosing around their deer feeding stump, licking up the few stray grains the deer had missed. The animal didn't appear overly steady on its feet, which is normally something that would worry her in case the animal was diseased. However, when it ran into the tree in front of it, she knew something was horribly wrong. She called to the animal on a whim, but she was not prepared for what she saw— two dead white eyes staring back through the darkness. She called her husband, and the two of them cautiously followed the animal for a half of a mile or so only to discover it was a stray dog. The dog was in horrible shape. He was malnourished (only sixty pounds in contrast to the ninety-eight or so he should have been) and was covered in briars and ticks. And then there were those two white eyes.

The couple put the dog in their barn and provided five small meals a day to begin to rebuild his strength. All of the ads they placed in local papers went unanswered, and no one in the local community knew who he was or what had brought him to their little town. As the woman described it, they lived in one of the poorest counties of the poorest state in the country, and animals were a fairly expendable commodity. There were no county veterinarians or local humane societies. Animal shelters were a luxury that their community could not afford. Strays were expected to fend for themselves or die, since there was no extra food or resources that could be spared for non-humans. Fortunately for the dog, the woman could not bear to leave him without assistance, so after some research she found an animal rescue in Chicago that agreed to send a volunteer to pick up the dog and help find him a good home. While waiting for the rescue volunteer, this kind woman made a lovely picture book that chronicled his painful beginnings. When Peggy eventually saw the dog's picture and learned that it was officially blind, she immediately wanted him. As she describes it, "It was my motherly instincts." The dog and the picture book soon became Peggy's

Although Peggy didn't know much about having a blind dog, she soon learned that dogs don't view a disability such as blindness as a big deal. It just is. Peggy's new canine friend didn't wonder why he was blind, or even stop to think that he was any different from any other dog. This was just his life, and he was happy to live it to its fullest. After changing the dog's name from Stevie the Wonder Dog to Bobby Lee, the family found a happy rhythm. At the time, they lived in a second floor condo in Evanston Illinois, making navigating the stairs a top priority. The "step" command was a natural for Bobby Lee, and he immediately started prancing when the command was given, knowing that a step of some sort was inevitable. A second necessary command was "watch it," which, despite the irony of issuing such an ill-named command to a visually impaired dog, meant to veer a different direction to avoid colliding with something. Bobby Lee soon learned how to find his way through the house by following the walls, and Peggy soon discovered that a collar can easily become snagged on passing items as a blind dog navigates through a house. Bobby Lee became incredibly resourceful, using sounds and smells to compensate for his loss of sight.

Ever since Peggy and her husband had met, their plan had been to move to Washington State. It was their dream. He would enjoy early retirement, and she could follow her heart. They found a wonderful home with land for the pups to run and play. The bottom of the lot was fenced, allowing Alex room for his favorite activity, fetch. Needless to say, Bobby Lee did not excel at that game. Bobby Lee was more laid-back— southern gentleman, if you will. He was unassuming, and would happily just sit by his people and accept an occasional scratch when offered. While he thoroughly enjoyed lounging on the porch, it soon became clear to Peggy that Bobby Lee needed an activity at which he could excel. There is definitely something to the old dog trainer's adage that every dog needs a job. Alex's job was chasing that ball around his yard. Bobby Lee was unemployed. And so began the search for something for Bobby Lee to do with his time.

Unsure where to start, Peggy wrote her local newspaper looking for leads for activities for Bobby Lee. Through the newspaper she learned about the Delta Society and the possibility of therapy dog work. "But could a blind dog do that?" wondered Peggy. With no where else to turn, Peggy looked through her telephone book to research trainers, and then registered for an upcoming workshop. Although one would think that training a blind dog to become a therapy dog would be a challenge, this was not the case, for Bobby Lee was a natural. Other than perfecting his leash walking skills, he only needed to learn the "down" command and he was ready to test. The only difficult aspect of the actual test was walking past a neutral dog. Since Bobby Lee was unable to read the normal canine communication skills of body language, glances, and gestures, he was dependent on what he learned from the sounds the other dog was making. If the other dog ignored him and walked on by, so did Bobby Lee. If the other dog turned toward him and barked, so did Bobby Lee. He was clearly a reactor when it came to other dogs since he had no ability to read the situation differently and to come to his own conclusions about the interaction. Despite this one weakness, he mastered all the other elements; he was comfortable with loud noises, crowding, being bumped, etc. Pretty good for a therapy dog; blind or sighted.

As Bobby Lee and Peggy began their work as a therapy dog team at a local hospital's pediatric unit, they soon discovered potential problems. Being a large dog (now close to a hundred pounds), it was challenging to maneuver in the cramped quarters of hospital rooms. Bobby Lee would become anxious as he struggled to determine what he was bumping into in the tiny hospital rooms, and Peggy struggled to assist him to find his way while not endangering any expensive equipment. Once an opening was available for them to work on the chemical dependency unit, they quickly took it, and found it to be a much better fit. Bobby Lee was able to wait in the community room with Peggy while the patients came to him. The patients loved the visits, and Bobby Lee was able to feel comfortable in the roomier setting. During these visits, his blindness always comes up. It's hard to miss that Bobby Lee is blind, and what a wonderful lesson for the patients. Peggy carries his storybook to tell his visitors his life story. Many of them are struggling with having to deal with a life that is less than ideal. Struggles and difficulties loom ahead, and many have no idea how they will navigate their new world. Following a visit from Bobby Lee, it is common to hear a patient say, "Well, if Bobby Lee can have a job and be productive despite his blindness and difficult start, then so can I."

Just when things were becoming more routine, Peggy noticed that Bobby Lee's right eye was beginning to swell, and he was beginning to paw at it, indicating that it was bothering him. Visits to the vet confirmed that Bobby Lee was suffering from glaucoma secondary to his cataracts. Despite several months of efforts to control the pressure through eye drops and other procedures, it soon became clear that Bobby Lee needed to have his right eye removed. As is typical in times of trauma and change, Bobby Lee's humans had the more difficult time dealing with this new disfigurement. Bobby Lee took it in stride, and it didn't have any significant impact on his work.

Bobby Lee continues to visit at the chemical dependency unit, but now also engages in other community work such as visiting the local health fair and grade school as well. During one such visit to a group of third graders, Bobby Lee received a note penned by a compassionate young boy. It simply read, "I'm sorry you are blind. If I could give you my eyes so you could see in color, I would." Bobby Lee has also received countless pictures, thoughtfully drawn by his young friends. Each shows Bobby Lee missing an eye, as the little artists do their best to accurately portray their canine visitor.

For the most part, Bobby Lee's blindness does not get in the way, but when it does, he depends on his human partner, Peggy, to help him through. On one such occasion, Peggy and Bobby Lee were volunteering at a Christmas auction. They were one of several teams working the event, and the tables were close together. Bobby Lee kept bumping into tables and people, and he had finally just had enough. He sat down in confusion and refused to move, unsure where to find a clearing. After some coaxing,

Peggy was able to lead him out of the maze of tables, chairs, and people. Bobby Lee depends on Peggy to navigate through life's challenging spots. Over the years, a deep friendship has formed between them, and this dependency is now mutual. At one point during my interview with Peggy she confided, "I think a part of me will die, too, when he passes away."

Once Peggy discovered the joy that Bobby Lee brought, and as she learned that it is not difficult to care for a special needs dog, she and her husband decided to adopt another blind dog named Danni. She is now seven months old, and is Bobby Lee's best friend. Before the adoption, a thorough veterinary exam revealed that little Danni had had lesions on her corneas when she was younger which were never properly treated. They later ruptured and caused blindness. Peggy hopes that, eventually, Danni will be able to become a therapy dog and carry on Bobby Lee's legacy when it comes time for him to retire. But for now she and Bobby Lee are content to wrestle and play, oblivious that there is anything different about them.

Peggy describes Bobby Lee as completely unassuming and undemanding. He's a good sized chocolate lab (she now describes him as "milk chocolate" as he begins to gray around his muzzle and eye). They live a simple life, yet one that is truly appreciated. The highlight of their day is the unleashed walk through the woods together. Peggy has learned a lot from Bobby Lee, she tells me. He is her soul mate. She has never been so close to a dog, nor has she ever learned so much. Through watching him, she has become more grounded. She used to live and work in the big city. Her husband used to refer to it as the "concrete canyon" as thousand of people rushed past, bumping into one another with no thought but for where they needed to be. She dreamed of a much slower-paced life with clean air, mountains, and evergreens. Now that dream is her reality, and she has learned that there is more to life than material things. By watching how resourceful Bobby Lee is in getting through life, she has learned to appreciate a more natural and resourceful way of living as well. Before, she was content to depend on things just because they were available and easier. Now she challenges this, and doesn't just take the easier path because it exists. Her dream now is to someday have a sanctuary for disabled animals—dogs, chickens, and the like. This is something she never would have considered in her past life as a city dweller. Helping others (both human and animal) has become her way of contributing to this world.

Although those who see Bobby Lee say he has a disability, Bobby Lee does not view himself as different from any other dog. He doesn't focus on himself, but only enjoys each moment he has been given. When Bobby Lee bumps into something during his day-to-day life, he simply stops, shakes it off, and finds another way. No need to fret or despair; he just takes it in stride and keeps focused on his goal. If only all of us could manage obstacles and challenges in this manner, imagine how simple life could be.

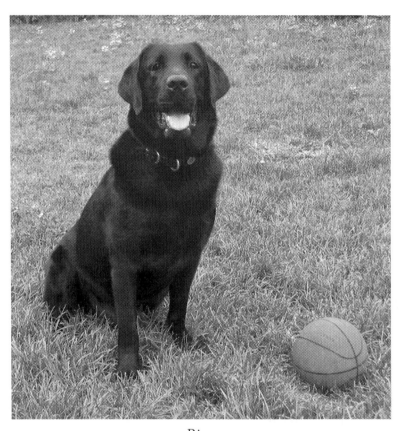

Rigo
*Photo by Diana McQuarrie*

# Chapter Ten
# Rigo

*We long for an affection*
*altogether ignorant of our*
*faults. Heaven has accorded*
*this to us in the uncritical*
*canine attachment.*

—George Eliot

Each dog on this earth has enormous potential. Each comes to us with individual talents, characteristics, and resources that are unique to that animal, and when perfectly matched to the task at hand, that dog can work miracles. In America, we love our pets. As a nation we spend an unfathomable amount of dollars on our furry four-legged friends. We have countless articles of clothing, boutiques, bakeries, spas, and the like available to ensure that our dear pets are dutifully pampered in ways that humans desire. Unfortunately, these same seemingly pampered pups are often unintentionally neglected in the very ways that matter most. By viewing a dog through human eyes and believing that he or she thinks and desires in the same fashion as humans, we often fail to see and appreciate dogs for who they really are. The majority of Americans are incredibly busy, leaving little time to devote to their canine friends. The unintended result is that the majority of dogs in America live a life in which their full potential remains untapped. While many of these pampered pups may very well enjoy a life of human leisure, their human family members have never really considered what their pets could become should someone take the time to really get to know them for who they are and discover and hone their innate gifts.

On the other end of the continuum lies a group of dogs

that is specifically bred and raised to take full advantage of their special talents and gifts. They are guide dogs for the blind. On the surface one might mistakenly think that these dogs are only tools to assist humans, without regard to the wants and desires of the individual canines. Each dog is purposefully bred for the very characteristics humans have determined to be most helpful for the task at hand, and each puppy is then carefully trained from puppyhood to assume a noble profession chosen by humans; the canines' destinies are already prescribed before their true personalities and traits are fully developed. At first glance it can sound cold and calculating, yet upon closer inspection, one finds a much more compassionate intent with a genuine desire for matching and ensuring that each and every little pup finds the perfect setting in which his or her talents can thrive. This is the story of Rigo, a very special little pup bred, raised, and trained through the Guide Dogs for the Blind in San Rafael, California.

The date was July 13, 2002. A perfect black Labrador retriever was born with his littermates, after selective breeding and the evaluation of genetic inheritances ensured that he qualified for the perfection of performance demanded from a guide dog. Everything was perfect, and he passed the special aptitude tests that demonstrated that he possessed the superior natural tendencies inherent in a guide dog. At seven weeks of age, he was entrusted to a carefully selected, experienced puppy-raising family that would provide the necessary environment Rigo required to develop into a guide. It was the family's responsibility to ensure that Rigo learned all the necessary life skills to assume the important job of guiding a blind person. While he had no idea what his future held, his new foster family was well aware of the importance of a solid foundation. He would need to be so reliable that his blind person would be able to experience the independence of a sighted person, living free from the apprehension of impending danger—quite a big responsibility for such a little pup. With this foster family he would learn about love, family, attachment, manners, and the world—the good and the scary. He would learn to ride buses, lie quietly under tables in restaurants, to ignore squirrels, manage loud noises, and trust his people—so many lessons.

Rigo learned these lessons well, and at fourteen months of age he made the trip back to the Guide Dogs for the Blind in California to begin his formal harness training. After acing his six months of harness training, he was matched with a gentleman who had been blind for many years and was receiving his fifth guide dog. Rigo succeeded in all other areas of his short life, but for some reason he just couldn't seem to conquer the task of relieving himself on command (guide dogs are taught to "do their business" when told on a regular schedule to accommodate the blind person's accessibility and opportunity to take their dogs outside). Despite all the training and resources invested in Rigo, he didn't quite make the perfect grade required by Guide Dogs, and another guide dog was chosen to partner with the blind man. Guide Dogs decided that an alternative career would be the best choice for Rigo; an expensive decision, but a true testimony to the compassion and humaneness of the Guide Dogs for the Blind. Rigo was returned to his puppy raiser, and she was allowed to make the decision on a future in which Rigo's talents and training would be best utilized. Rigo was flown home from California to the woman who had lovingly raised him. After much soul searching, she decided to place him with her friend, Diana.

Diana had been a dog lover all her life. She had had a dog for as long as she could remember, and at the time of her friend's phone call to discuss adopting Rigo, she already had three dogs of her own. Her life had been forever changed when at the tender age of eight, she read a book entitled, *First Lady of the Seeing Eye,* by Morris Frank and Blake Clark. That book opened her eyes to the incredible work of guide dogs. From that day on, she dreamed of volunteering as a puppy raiser for future guide dogs, and she set a goal to have a career that would utilize dogs to help others. Her dream eventually came true when she and her husband, Ken, were able to volunteer for The Seeing Eye of Morristown, New Jersey.[4] Ken and Diana took in puppies, lovingly bringing up little balls of fur and skillfully working and training with them each day so they would grow up to be someone's cherished partner and friend. It was tremendously rewarding, and Diana continued to be involved with the guide dog community when she and her husband moved to Colorado in 2000. With demanding job responsibilities and three dogs of her own, she no longer raised guide dog puppies herself, but dedication for the work remained an important part of her heart. Diana's journey in animal-assisted therapy began with a defining moment in 1991, when she and Ken fell in love with an adorable seven-week-old golden retriever named Shana, whom they lovingly trained from puppyhood. When Shana was four years old and had begun to mellow with age (her field bloodlines made her rather energetic in her younger years), Diana began to explore the world of animal-assisted therapy. It was a perfect match for them both. Soon they were registered Pet Partners through the Delta Society and were visiting in hospitals, schools, and nursing homes in addition to giving presentations about the human-animal bond.

When Shana was ten years old, Diana discovered that she had a maxillary fibrosarcoma, a potentially deadly form of cancer, in her upper right jaw. Diana pulled her from therapy work and began treatment in earnest. Thankfully, she caught the cancer early, and with surgery and good treatment Shana made a full recovery. It was then that Diana discovered Shana's true calling; working with oncology patients. Shana gave cancer patients something that others could not—the gift of understanding and hope. It was magical to watch. Diana eventually became the founder

---

4 The Seeing Eye is the pioneer guide dog school in the United States. Since 1929, the mission of The Seeing Eye has been to enhance the independence, dignity, and self-confidence of blind people through the use of seeing eye dogs.

and executive director of Denver Pet Partners, a Delta Society affiliate. Through Diana, human-animal teams throughout the Denver Metro area found a sense of community.

So was it any wonder that Rigo's puppy raiser thought of her friend Diana in May of 2004 when the dog was in need of a good home? Diana had retired Shana from therapy work in September 2003. While partnering with Shana in 2001, Diana had acquired a six-year-old chocolate lab, Gypsy, who was a retired field trial dog. Less than a year later, Gypsy's kennel-mate from the same breeder, Biskit, a yellow lab, retired from the show ring and also found a forever home with Diana. Diana then successfully did therapy work with her two Labrador retrievers, as well as with Shana. This met Shana's needs for a lighter work schedule as she neared retirement age. While she was able to match Gypsy and Biskit to settings to fit their unique talents and personalities, neither had the ability to visit in the complex settings that Shana had. Diana painfully watched Shana endure multiple illnesses in the year following her retirement. She survived a serious bout with Lyme disease which left her visually impaired and temporarily lame. She suffered a stroke which impacted her balance, and with increasingly advanced age, began suffering from benign tumorous lesions. It was painful for Diana to watch her dear partner suffer so, especially after the dog had given of herself so selflessly for many years.

Rigo was a welcome addition to Diana's life. Although her home was already full of canines and her emotions overwhelmingly preoccupied with the inevitable destiny of her ailing canine friend, Rigo was a dream come true. Diana's work with the Guide Dogs for the Blind had come full circle, as she embraced Rigo and worked with him to find his perfect fit in life.

At first Rigo wasn't sure what his role should be. "Diana must be blind," he likely surmised as he dutifully showed her curbs and steps to make sure his new human remained safe and wasn't harmed by unforeseen obstacles. However, in short time he figured out that his role wasn't to be a guide for Diana. Regardless, he stuck by her side at all times and ignored all others (just as he was trained to do in guide school), only to find that Diana patiently invited him to visit with others. It was a difficult transition from service dog thinking to therapy dog thinking. A service dog is trained to serve only one, while a therapy dog works with many. With time, Rigo welcomed his freedom to interact with others and began to settle into a comfortable partnership with Diana. But it wasn't until one autumn day that Rigo discovered his true work.

The day was September 16, 2005. Shana's health had continued to fail, and when her lung cancer metastasized to her other internal organs, Diana and Ken knew that the end of Shana's journey had come. In an effort to make her passing as dignified as possible, they chose home euthanasia and gently brought their cherished family member to a favorite spot where she always liked to lay and look out across the garden and backyard. Here they would spend their last moments on this earth together. They left the French doors to the back patio open so that the family dogs could come and go as they pleased. They knew what lay ahead would be difficult and painful and were unsure how their canine family members would choose to respond. This day was Shana's last day with her beloved family. One at a time, entirely by their own choosing, each lab lovingly came up to Shana as she was cradled in Diana's arms and said their good-byes by gently nosing Shana's mature gray muzzle. Gypsy, the chocolate lab, always intensely loyal and close by to Diana, then dutifully took her place directly two feet behind Diana. She could feel the depth of Diana's sorrow, and she sat behind her in silent support. Biskit, the beautiful yellow lab, quietly went to the family room where she lay on her favorite bed and silently observed all that was to take place. Rigo, still new to the family and an extremely sensitive dog, left the scene. He went to the front door and stared out the window. Observing Diana's pain and grief was overwhelming for him, and he didn't know what to do. As Shana breathed her last breath and Diana's deep sorrow was expressed in sobs, Rigo understood what his job on this earth was. It was not to bravely guide a blind person through life; it was to heal and protect Diana's heart. He instantly knew that she was more than his person, she was now his responsibility. He just knew.

From that moment forward the bond between Rigo and Diana deepened. Diana took Rigo everywhere with her. She needed him, and he now understood the importance of his role. He was no longer the guide dog who failed; he was now Diana's canine partner in life. His very presence provided incredible comfort to her, and he helped her to cope with the immensely painful loss of her beloved Shana. Together they have become a human-animal team to emulate. Rigo's special training and extensive socialization make him the ideal therapy dog. Nothing fazes him, and this allows him to enjoy settings that would induce stress in other therapy dogs. Together they now work in a wide variety of settings including an in-patient rehab unit in a large hospital, a mental health center for children who have suffered trauma and abuse, and at numerous speaking engagements to provide public education on the human-animal bond. He accompanies Diana as she teaches graduate school classes and conducts courses for healthcare professionals who wish to incorporate animal-assisted therapy into their own practices. In addition, Rigo is a demo dog for courses Diana teaches for those who wish to do therapy work with their pets. Lastly, Rigo is certified as a disaster relief dog with the Red Cross and is also a regular blood donor at a local animal emergency clinic.

On the day that I met Rigo and Diana, they had just finished assisting a therapist on the rehab unit at a large university hospital. Diana smiled as she told me how much she loves their Friday morning animal-assisted therapy sessions, for during these times they see the same patients on multiple occasions over two to three weeks. They get to witness the patients' progress and see the difference they are making in the patients' lives. During these sessions, she and Rigo assist in the therapy for patients who are recovering from various ailments such as burns on up to ninety percent of their bodies, strokes, brain injuries, and brain tumors. Rigo seems to know instinctively how to interact with each patient. When he is asked to tug on a rope to provide the necessary resistance to develop the patient's muscles, Diana watches in amazement as Rigo seems to know just how much pressure to exert for each patient, providing greater resistance for patients with more strength and minimal resistance to those who are more fragile. As we talked, Diana pulled out a baby blue felt vest that Rigo wears as he helps other patients develop their muscle coordination and language sequencing skills. Rigo waits patiently while the patients' follow the therapist's directions to place various colored felt shapes, letters, and numbers onto his felt vest.

Diana told me several stories about their work with these patients. One such patient had suffered a stroke. There was a vacant look in her eyes, the kind of look that let Diana know that her brain was not processing information correctly. But Rigo made a connection with this woman. Although holding eye contact is not a natural behavior for a dog (it is considered to be rude and aggressive in canine culture), Rigo has the ability to gently hold his gaze with his kind, soft eyes, and it was precisely this skill that allowed Rigo to profoundly connect with this woman in a way that no human had been able to do since her injury. On another occasion, Diana and Rigo were working with a woman who was suffering from an inoperable brain tumor. While patients with these kinds of situations frequently can not even remember their own children's name, this woman was able to remember Rigo's name each session. During their last session together, Diana gave the woman Rigo's business card so she could remember him. She lifted the card to her lips and gently kissed the card. She then said, "I love Rigo" as she was wheeled down the hallway to her room. That was the last time Diana ever saw that woman, but she knew she and Rigo had made a difference in her life.

Diana then told me about their work with burn patients. Outside of the hospital setting it would be highly unlikely that Diana would ever have had the opportunity to interact with someone in those circumstances. She spoke about the shame and embarrassment that these patients often feel due to their forever-changed appearance. They are incredibly self-conscious and normally don't want anyone to see their scarred faces, but they welcome a visit from Rigo. They know that Rigo sees past their scars and imperfections. Rigo unconditionally accepts them how they are. It is just the medicine they need to begin the healing.

Rigo and Diana also frequently visit in the school systems. They are ambassadors for the human-animal bond, and together they are the perfect team to educate children about respect for life, compassion, and what a well-trained dog is like. Many children in impoverished neighborhoods have never experienced the love and companionship that a dog can offer. Dogs with whom they have come in contact are often used for protection or are untrained. As a result, the children have not learned how to appropriately and safely interact with a dog, and have never experienced the life-changing bond that comes from forming a friendship with a well-trained canine. These children often leave these educational settings and return home to tell excited stories to their parents about their visit with the wonderful therapy dog. Diana smiled as she told me of numerous personal letters and hand-drawn pictures the students have sent to her and Rigo in appreciation. These mementos hold a special place in her heart, for they speak to the lasting difference their work is making in people's lives each day.

Diana then told me about a third setting in which she and Rigo work. It is a preschool for blind children. Visiting with Rigo provides an ideal opportunity for the children to learn about body parts, learn about touch, learn how to be safe around a dog, and experience what it feels like to walk beside a dog. Diana then pulled a harness from her bag that Rigo wears when they work with these children. The children can hold the harness and allow Rigo to guide them while Diana holds the leash and walks alongside. While the children are still too young to fully conceptualize the possibility of a guide dog, Diana and Rigo plant seeds that dogs can be wonderful partners in life.

The potential work settings are endless for Diana and Rigo. They regularly teach in various settings about therapy dog work and about the human-animal bond. Rigo serves as the consummate example of what every therapy dog can only hope to be someday. Although they have only been together as a team for a few years, you would never know by watching them work. They complement each other perfectly, providing opportunities for each other and touching lives in ways that would be impossible to achieve by themselves.

As my time with Rigo and Diana came to a close, her husband, Ken, joined us. I could not help but ask for his opinion as to how Rigo has changed Diana. Although Diana had thoughtfully answered all my questions, my heart told me that there was a deeper difference that Rigo has made in Diana's life. Ken did not hesitate even for a moment in his answer. "When Rigo's around, everything is all right with Diana," he said. He then went on to tell me that Diana always has to know where Rigo is around the house. "She isn't comfortable until she knows." Rigo has finally reached his full potential, as he fills a void in Diana's life. Although he was bred and raised to be a guide dog for a blind person, he found his true calling. In Diana he has found someone who truly appreciates his unique talents and characteristics and with whom he can partner to share these with others. Rigo now gives the gift of unconditional love and acceptance to those who need it most, while always remembering that his first responsibility is his human friend, Diana.

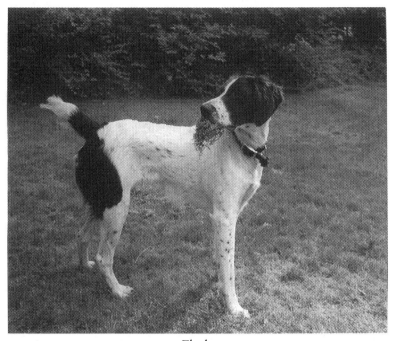

Flash
*Photo by Kathy Whitlock*

# Chapter Eleven
# Flash

*The average dog has one
request to all humankind.
Love me.*

—Helen Exley

Hospitals can be scary places. People who inhabit the beds are suffering from various ailments, and noisy, intimidating equipment rattles and clangs as white-clad employees push it down the long hallways. Conversations can be awkward as visitors and patients confront fear, discomfort, and, at times, mortality. Hospital employees are frequently harried as they struggle to juggle their daily tasks with the unexpected crises that are inherent with caring for the ill. Over the course of my work, it has not been uncommon to hear adults confess that they avoid hospitals at all costs. Even visiting a close friend or family member can be the source of great angst. In a place where conversations frequently encompass only the subjects of illness and problems, many simply choose not to go, trusting that their loved ones will be released home soon. Now, these same people are quick to admit that they should go visit or that they are well aware that their loved one may be lonely or would benefit from a visit, but they can't seem to muster the courage to surmount their own discomfort for the good of others.

This discomfort and apprehension is precisely why therapy dogs work miracles in hospital settings. When a therapy dog sets paw into a hospital, the topic of conversation quickly shifts from fears and problems to the enjoyment of the moment. Happier times and pleasant memories become the theme of conversation, and long lost smiles are seen once again. Even nurses and doctors take a break from the hustle and bustle of their hectic schedules to enjoy the moment. For patients, "What ifs" are temporarily forgotten as the focus shifts to "Remember when ...." With a therapy dog by one's side, even a person who previously was terribly uncomfortable and at a loss to begin a conversation in such a setting can suddenly forget the discomfort and focus on the needs of those who need a visit. Such is the story of Flash.

On March 30, 1999, Flash was born to a breeder in Washington State. He was mostly white with just a splash of brown on his head and hindquarters. A perfect little purebred German shorthaired pointer, he was only twenty-five pounds and four and a half months old when he first met his new family. He was specially chosen by Kathy and Doug for Doug's birthday present. While they had had dogs throughout their thirty-three-year marriage, this was to be Doug's first dog of his very own, and he had thought long and hard before deciding upon a German shorthair. He and Kathy had had German shorthair/lab mixes before, but Doug had settled upon a purebred this time—the perfect dog to accompany him on hunting trips.

Upon bringing Flash home to Fat Cat Ranch, Kathy and Doug began to enjoy his budding personality. He was amazingly playful and energetic; always running about. He would dash up the hill towards Canada, with only a "flash" of white to be seen. That's how Doug discovered the pup's perfect name, Flash Dogg of Fat Cat Ranch (the word "dog" is not allowed in official names for purebred canines registered with the American Kennel Club, so they decided to spell it "Dogg"). When Flash did sit still, he preferred to be a lap dog, loving to lounge with his new humans and be held. His sweet disposition was irresistible. Even the family cat, Spot, took a liking to Flash and the two became inseparable best friends. They could readily be found on the living room couch with Flash nuzzled up to Spot like a soft, cozy pillow. It didn't hurt that the orangey-tan and white Spot already viewed himself as a dog, and had a long history before Flash's arrival of insisting that he accompany the family on walks. He would lounge on the seat of Kathy's mother's walker or ride in the wheelbarrow atop a load of hay. Before long, Flash joined Spot in following Doug and Kathy around the ranch as they fed the cows, tended to fences, and completed all the many chores that come with owning property.

Doug had always loved dogs, although his family never had one when he was growing up. He and Kathy met in high school, and soon Doug was a regular over at her house, playfully saying he was really coming just to visit her Great Dane. Kathy, on the other hand, had been raised around animals all her life. Her first dog was a spaniel that she received as a gift for her first birthday. When she and Doug married, animals were a given in their relationship; cats, dogs, cows, and even a horse all took up residence at their ranch. Kathy had dutifully trained the couple's many prior dogs, but decided this time that it was Doug's responsibility to take the lead on training Flash. So off they went to class, with Kathy supportively on the sideline. While Flash loved to run and play with his classmates, attending to the obedience lessons was not his forte. Despite his lack of focus, he passed the class, but not before picking up a certificate for the "most improved" dog in class. Although technically successful, that class ended his academic career since the instructor feared that Flash would view any advanced training such as agility as an excuse to run around and have fun rather than pay attention to the lessons.

With basic training behind them, life became their teacher. Each morning began with Doug calling for Flash as they made their way to the old black Acura for the trip to Mr. Doug's Eatery for breakfast (Kathy playfully pointed out the irony of the name when telling me this part of the story, since her husband has no relationship to the origin of the diner's name). When making their way down the quarter-mile driveway, Doug would open the moon roof until they reached the road so Flash could stand on the console and stick his head out to see the view, his ears flapping in the gentle breeze. Once at the diner, Doug enjoyed a quiet breakfast while catching up with the morning paper or visiting with acquaintances in the quiet little town. It was a cherished ritual for this retired man and his dog, as Flash waited patiently for Doug to finish his coffee and make his way back to the car seat that Flash kept warm for the trip back home. Once home they took a long leisurely walk across the beautiful Puget Sound preserves, dotted with diverse flora and fauna. Although Doug walked four to five miles each time, Flash added countless miles to the route as he scurried from thing to thing, his nose held close to the ground looking for anything of interest; making the most of his time in nature. Both came home from these journeys refreshed and ready to enjoy the comfort of the couch. As the years passed, Flash began to settle, and the characteristic freckles and small spots seen on German shorthairs began to appear. He filled out to his present tall, long-legged, fifty-five-pound stature; with longer feathered fur on his legs, tail, ears, and belly. Some say he looks like a tall springer spaniel, while others question if he is part Dalmatian. However, no one ever questioned that he grew into an incredibly sweet dog. Flash naturally developed the ability to turn on and off his energy, making him the perfect couch potato as well as the ideal outdoor enthusiast.

Although Flash was technically Doug's dog, no dog can live in the home without becoming close with Kathy. Flash was always the first to notice when Kathy was feeling under the weather, and he quickly responded by lying in the bed or on the couch with his head lovingly in her lap to offer support or comfort. It was Kathy who patiently taught Flash to fetch (not an easy trick to learn when one thinks it far more fun to simply grab the ball and run around with it as a prize). With time, Kathy had Flash promptly returning the ball and eagerly dropping it in anticipation for the much appreciated treat. It was at some point during these years that Kathy first considered Flash as a potential therapy dog. She had first heard about the wonderful work that the Delta Society (located near her hometown) was doing at a local hospital. She had even considered working with her lab/German shorthair mix, Arrow. He was a beautiful black dog with gorgeous white markings on his chest and big floppy ears. A striking dog, but Kathy ultimately decided it was asking too much of Arrow to begin a career at the ripe old age of ten.

So her focus shifted to Flash, and she began to fine tune his training. Trainers suggested that in order to effectively train a potential therapy dog, she should take Flash to the local grocery store parking lot to visit with patrons as they neared the store. She eagerly explained to visitors her efforts to better socialize Flash for his future career, and they were more than willing to assist in the project. Flash loved these outings, and enjoyed it when people approached him to visit. And Kathy soon discovered that Flash was a very different dog when working; much more calm and focused. In an effort to see how Flash would respond to formal visiting, Kathy brought Flash with her into the assisted living center where she was a regular volunteer. Flash was a natural.

When the time came to take the therapy dog exam, Flash was a champ. He seemed to know instinctively just how to complete each exercise and how to best read each scenario. However, he did let his true personality shine through when he characteristically refused to sit on command during the test. Flash did what Kathy had seen him do so many times before. He simply pretended not to hear her. After much persistence on Kathy's part, Flash complied with a loud sigh. In many ways, Flash is simply a big kid testing to see if he *really* has to obey. When Kathy told me this part of her story, she quickly offered a possible explanation for Flash's behavior. She was extremely nervous that day during the test, and Flash may have felt the need to "stand guard." However, I couldn't help but notice this theme of Flash gently showing his own opinion, which kept showing up in many aspects of Flash's story and seemed to be better explained as an endearing part of his personality.

As official Delta Society Pet Partners, Kathy and Flash began their visits to the nearby hospital. Now it is important to note here that Kathy has historically avoided visiting friends and loved ones in hospitals. Despite working for many years in a doctor's office located within a hospital and even working directly in a hospital during her college years, she remained safely tucked away in the office setting and had managed to avoid having to interact much with patients. She remained uncomfortable and unsure what to say. However, with Flash by her side, gone were the fears and her apprehension of hospitals. Flash was the perfect topic of conversation, and paved the way to countless conversations about patients' and staff members' pets. The pet partners began their work on the first floor, visiting in the many waiting rooms for the x-ray department, surgery, outpatient laboratory, and intensive care. These were busy days, with Flash and Kathy visiting forty to fifty people over the course of a couple of hours. The environment was sometimes thick with tension due to the personal fears and sadness experienced by the visitors. Not everyone wanted a visit, and sensing who did and who would prefer to be left alone was a skill that Flash quickly developed. On occasion, a visitor would simply raise his newspaper or look away in response to seeing Flash, and with time, Flash learned to walk on by. Flash became an expert at determining who had family pets and who might appreciate a visit. Pet owners seemed to enjoy being spotted by Flash and the resultant visit. One of Flash's favorite places was the intensive care unit, since the staff members were always so happy to see him. The dog provided the perfect stress relief for them in their hectic work day, and he was even allowed to visit select patients in the unit with doctor's permission. On one occasion, Kathy saw two women, clearly distraught, sitting on the floor, talking, outside one of the rooms. They seemed very worried about their mother, who was in the adjacent hospital room. As Kathy and Flash approached, the women suddenly invited Flash to join them. Sensing their worry, Flash laid his head in one of the women's laps and settled in to enjoy the time. Kathy sat beside them, allowing them to sit in peaceful silence with Flash. Just when Kathy thought Flash had drifted off to sleep, he would slowly open one eye or gently thump his tail to signal to his partner he was just enjoying the moment. Near the end of the visit the women mentioned how much their mother loved dogs and would like a visit when she was feeling better. Kathy quickly explained the necessity of therapy dogs having doctor's permission and explained how they could arrange that for their mother. As they stood to leave, both women were smiling, their mood markedly improved despite the gravity of their mother's condition. Flash was just the diversion they needed to better face their situation.

Flash soon became a favorite on the pediatric unit as well. With strict rules against jumping onto beds, Kathy taught Flash how to carefully step onto a bed with the patient's permission to snuggle for a bed visit with his tiny patients. Hospitals can be tremendously scary places to children. Watching television with Flash by their side was just the medicine needed to lift the spirits of these little patients. Children tell Flash about their own pets, or simply enjoy the touch of his silky fur. Parents are grateful for a happy moment, sometimes whispering to Kathy that this was the first time the child smiled or said a word in this scary setting. On one of these visits, Flash and Kathy met a child who had been bitten by a dog. The bite had become infected, requiring hospitalization. Cautiously entering the room at the child's mother's invitation, Kathy was sensitive to the possibility that the tiny patient might now be fearful of dogs. This fear soon vanished as the child's eyes lit up at the sight of Flash's doggy smile and wagging tail.

On another occasion, Kathy and Flash were walking down the hallway of the pediatric unit, when Kathy knocked on the door of a young boy's room. She quietly asked if the boy would like a visit from Flash only to be surprised by the response of an older woman by the boy's bedside, "I don't know about John, but his grandmother sure would." Flash and Kathy happily entered the room, eager to meet John and his grandmother, when John quickly exclaimed, "I know Flash!" He went on to explain that he had met Flash when the pet partners had come to his school just a few months earlier. He told his mother and grandmother all about their visit to his school and everything he learned that day. As Kathy and Flash gathered their things to leave following the visit, John's mom thanked Kathy, saying that this was the first time John had seemed happy or smiled since coming to the hospital the day before.

One of Kathy's favorite places to visit in the hospital is the rehabilitation unit because of the variety it provides. In this unit, it is frequently Flash's role to motivate patients to stand, exercise their limbs, or perform various exercises. Flash enjoys walking with his patients, and he seems to know just the ideal speed for their impairment, pacing himself to the client's gait. In addition, he has perfected knowing his right from his left, and readily makes the correct turn at Kathy's verbal request. For some, Flash is the needed incentive to rise from their wheelchairs and take the lap around the room to exercise and speed their recovery. For some, asking a patient to stand, throw the ball for Flash to retrieve, and then sit back down provides the same physical movements that these same patients refuse to do without the interaction of a therapy dog. Flash's patients have been known to stand longer than the required time out of pure enjoyment of watching Flash run after the ball. On one such occasion, Flash was working with an elderly gentleman. The therapist was having a difficult time getting him to stand for the necessary five seconds. The gym was far too crowded for Flash to successfully retrieve a ball, so Kathy was challenged to get creative. She quickly thought of the five bones that are on his therapy dog vest symbolizing his five years of service—three on one side and two on the other. At Kathy's suggestion, the therapist asked the gentleman to stand and count the bones on Flash's vest before sitting back down. Once standing, the man began to count; one... two ... three. He then chuckled as Kathy maneuvered Flash to change positions, so the gentleman could count the remaining two bones—four ... five. As a result of his laughter and enjoyment of the activity, the man actually stood for ten seconds or more!

Flash also enjoys being brushed as stroke patients practice their hand movements through this repetitive movement. He then rolls over to encourage them to continue their excellent work on his belly. Other stroke patients enjoy reminiscing about past pets, which provides the needed mental stimulation to aid their recall and memory. Such seemingly simple exercises often have staggering results.

In addition to their work at the hospital, Flash and Kathy enjoy visiting (with other Delta Society Pet Partner teams) the local third grade classes at all the schools in her district of approximately twenty thousand children. Together, they visit weekly for over two months in order to provide this opportunity to all the third graders. One of Kathy's favorite parts of visiting in the schools is the letters of appreciation they write to her and Flash (see Figure 1), for they show how much the children enjoy the visits. In preparation, the children read *Rosy the Visiting Dog* to better understand the role of a therapy dog. The coordinator then conducts a short presentation about the components of the therapy dog test, grooming requirements, etc. On occasion, the dogs express their impatience with the lecture, lying down with a loud sigh and a thump. Although Flash clearly loves this activity, Kathy has learned that three classes of children in a day are all he can manage. It is enjoyable, but also stressful and exhausting, leaving him looking for the door as a sign it is time to call it a day.

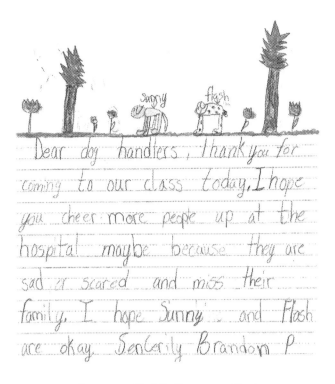

Dear dog handlers, Thank you for coming to our class today, I hope you cheer more people up at the hospital maybe because they are sad or scared and miss their family, I hope Sunny and Flash are okay. SenGerily Brandon P

Figure 1 Child's Letter to Flash

As I listened to Kathy's story, I found it hard to believe that she was once painfully uncomfortable interacting with people who were suffering from some ailment. She now seemed so incredibly confident as she rattled on about the many settings in which she and Flash visit and about the countless patients who have been changed by meeting Flash. Puzzled, I asked for further clarification to ensure that I had indeed understood this transformation correctly. She gently reminded me that this change was all because of Flash. It was because of Flash's comfort and ease with people that she is now comfortable as well. She gave the example of a ceramics class that she teaches at a local assisted living facility. While she had previously only interacted with the residents who took her class, Flash has encouraged her to meet new residents who might benefit from a kind word or from someone listening to their stories. Flash has a way of reminding her to look beyond her natural comfort level to see all the people who are around her. And, in so doing, she lost her own fear somewhere along the road.

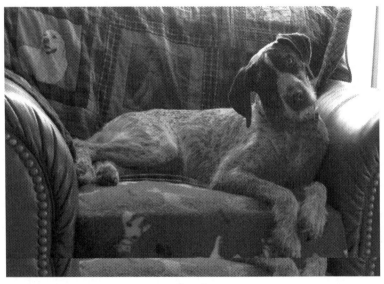

Annie
*Photo by Mary Beacon*

# Chapter Twelve
# Annie

*The one absolutely unselfish*
*friend that man can have in*
*this selfish world, the one that*
*never deserts him, the one that*
*never proves ungrateful or*
*treacherous, is his dog.*

—George Graham Vest

It seems that throughout one's life there are distinct chapters. All of us had the childhood chapter and most had the high school chapter, but from that point forward, the chapters frequently differ from person to person. As children we dream about how our lives will turn out; we dream about what chapters we will write in the story that will become our lives. When I was very young, I dreamed of being a doctor. I made wheelchairs out of cardboard boxes, wooden Tinker Toy parts, and empty paper towel rolls, and I created electrocardiogram machines out of boxes, adding machine paper, and string. My dolls and teddy bears dutifully stared straight ahead with their button eyes as I wrapped them in Ace bandages, gave them my candy "medicine" or "shocked" them back to life after yelling, "Clear!" and imitating the emergency room drama I had witnessed on my favorite seventies television show, *Emergency*. My mother played along by embroidering "Dr. Teri" on hand sewn strips of old sheets she transformed into hospital linens for my tiny patients. All of this was rehearsal for the medical chapter I expected to be part of my adult life.

As my high school chapter came to an end, I explored entering nursing school, only to decide to take a few years off and move to Colorado. After exploring several entry-level jobs within the medical field, I soon learned that blood and other bodily fluids were really quite disgusting to me, thereby forcing me to rethink the upcoming chapters in my life. Other preplanned chapters were marriage and children, so as I abandoned my previous career plans, I threw myself into writing the domestic chapter. During this period in my life I began to truly understand that life has a way of changing the best of plans, forcing us to adapt and embrace creative writing as we pen the chapters that are our lives. Tragedy, loss, and immaturity all forced twists and turns in my road of life. Who I thought I would be when I was a young child dreaming about my future is nothing like who I have become. Yet, like a best-selling novel, it is the unexpected plot twist and the surprise ending that engage the avid reader. Being a therapist and writer are far from the medical career path I foresaw for myself, yet I now realize these professions are the perfect fit for my gifts and who I truly am. And, while I always had a deep love for dogs, I never dreamed as a child that these joyous creatures would take such a central place in my personal and professional life. Although the uncertainty and harshness of life shape us all, it is up to each of us how we use these themes and story lines. As I ripen with age, I am no longer writing my life from a previously penned outline, but am curious and open to what the next chapter brings. It was at a similar juncture in Mary's life that we met, and she told me the story of Annie.

Mary and her husband, Jay, met in the early eighties. Although they both worked for the same company, it was their love of dogs and art that brought them together. A few years earlier, Jay had been in a tragic car accident that had crushed his spinal cord and left him with limited use of his legs. Yet despite his limitations, Jay remained extremely active, playing golf weekly and even managing to walk for short distances with the help of a cane even though professionals had cautioned that he would never walk again.

Jay was the love of Mary's life. He was perfect for her in every way, and he had a way of making her laugh and forget the worries of the world like no other was able to do. Theirs was the perfect chapter. So when the time came for Mary and Jay to decide upon the ideal family dog, it was no surprise that it was done in a playful and joyously humorous way. Jay wanted a big dog, and Mary had her heart set on a dog with "whiskers." After significant research regarding which breeds contained both of these traits, they decided upon a German wirehaired pointer, a breed with a wire-like coat and unique facial furnishings. "There is just something about the bushy eyebrows and beard that I love!" said Mary with a chuckle as she proceeded to tell me the potential perils of choosing a dog while knowing nothing of the breed's temperament. Lucky for Mary and Jay, they soon fell in love with the breed's personality as well and were taken with the intelligence that is characteristic of the breed.

They named their new puppy Ada. Soon Mary and Jay were enjoying obedience classes and dog shows, and it was then that Jay got the idea to train Ada to be his helper dog. Before long, Ada was skillfully retrieving any item to which Jay pointed. When out in public, Jay would playfully brag that he had the smartest dog in the world. And when challenged to prove this, Jay would then point and say, "Ada, bring me my keys." Ada would then disappear into the other room and return with Jay's keys dangling from her mouth, to the delight of onlookers. Jay would continue the antics, asking Ada to retrieve all kinds of items as Mary laughed, knowing that Ada was simply picking up whatever item at which Jay pointed. As the years went by, additional German wirehaired pointers and terriers joined the family. One of Jay's favorites was a wonderful Irish terrier named Conan the Barbarian. It became a common neighborhood sight for Jay to get out his three-wheeled bike, hook a dog to each side, and take off for a long bike ride, or to witness Mary in one of Jay's extra wheelchairs and Jay in his own wheelchair as each took a dog and enjoyed a lively wheelchair race down the quarter mile cul-de-sac. Mary laughed as she reminisced about these races, realizing now how wonderfully naive they were of the potential dangers of such antics. This was clearly one of Mary's favorite chapters in her life.

Then almost fifteen years after the chapter began, the story took an unexpected turn and a more painful chapter commenced. It was late winter of 2004, and Mary had just returned from a wonderful trip to New York with her sister to show her sister's smooth fox terrier in the Westminster Kennel Club Dog Show. As Mary was in the other room unpacking her things from travel, she heard her husband heating up a Stouffers TV dinner. As she entered the kitchen, he mentioned that he didn't feel well, so she helped him to the bedroom and into their bed when she saw it; one side of his face suddenly fell. She knew instantly that he had suffered a stroke. As she reached for the phone to call the ambulance, Jay began his protest. He hated hospitals. He had been incredibly healthy since the fateful car accident, and he did not want to return to hospitals and all the poking and prodding that they entail. But despite his objections, the paramedics came, and he was whisked away.

The weeks ahead were some of the most difficult for Mary. She spent most of the time at the hospital. Since the weather was permissible, she packed Conan, Gizmo (a German wirehair) and Sketch (a smooth fox terrier) into the van each morning with their beds and would run out to the parking lot to care for them and let them stretch their legs as she took a break from her bedside vigil. Their presence was a blessing to her as her heart was heavy with worry about Jay, and they could feel that something was terribly wrong as they licked away Mary's tears.

As Jay's condition improved, he was moved to the progressive care unit. Despite his physical improvements, he was uncharacteristically combative and angry. He hated being in the hospital, and he was angry with Mary for making the call that put him in the predicament. He was now suffering from aphasia, which was cruelly impairing his ability to produce and comprehend language. Angry outbursts were now an everyday occurrence. On one occasion Mary brought items and pictures from home, hoping to help Jay with his language skills and to lift his spirits, only to have Jay rip each picture in anger. But when he saw the picture of Conan, he only feigned ripping the picture, but then stealthily hid it under his blanket to admire at a later time. Wisely, Mary pretended she didn't see the hidden picture lest he rip it up as well.

As the weeks progressed, Jay was able to move to the rehabilitation unit. He agreed to this move under protest and with two requests: that his dog could visit and that Mary could bring him food from home. Mary decided to bring a home cooked meal to him each night. There in the progressive care unit a little westie with a local affiliate of the Delta Society came to visit and Mary first learned about animal-assisted activities and the work of therapy dogs. Seeing the difference this little dog's presence made, the hospital personnel told Mary that should she obtain medical clearance from her veterinarian, should she follow established rules, and should Conan pass a temperament test, they would allow her to bring Jay's favorite canine buddy into the hospital for nightly visits. Upon hearing this, Mary's vet quickly prepared the necessary documents and Conan was soon approved. Conan was the only one able to bring a smile of joy to Jay's face during these difficult weeks.

Every evening at five o'clock, Mary left Jay's side to return home, cook dinner, and return with a homemade meal for Jay, with Conan at her side. The usually full of mischief Conan was uncharacteristically well behaved, seemingly aware of the special hospital privileges he was receiving. Together Conan and Jay would lie side by side from five to nine o'clock each night with Mary close at hand, enjoying the moments. Mary would then leave for home at 9:00 p.m. only to return by three o'clock the next morning to make sure she was there when Jay first opened his eyes. As Mary and Conan walked the halls to and from Jay's room, other hospital patients and visitors began to ask for a visit as well. On one evening a woman on a gurney insisted that the orderly stop immediately. She would not allow the orderly to proceed until she was able to visit with Conan. These were powerful moments for Mary, as she began to witness the healing effects a dog can have on the human soul. Each evening Jay looked forward to his cherished visits from Conan as they snuggled together watching television or chatting with Mary. These were treasured respites from the medical worries and trepidations.

Eventually the day came that Jay was able to return home. The happiness was short lived, for tragically, Jay suffered from a hemorrhagic stroke three weeks later. This stroke caused extensive bleeding within his brain. Again, Mary called the paramedics, and once at the hospital she learned that he would most likely not survive. One of Jay's biggest fears was that of dying in a hospital. Respectful of this, Mary and the hospital staff worked quickly to move him back home with hospice care for his final days. Once home he was in a coma-like state, unable to move or communicate. Mary's siblings came to be with her to help, and on a couple of special occasions, Jay squeezed her hand to let her know that he knew she was there. It was the most incredibly difficult forty-eight hours as Mary enjoyed each moment she had left with her dear husband. Conan, Gizmo, and Sketch seemed to sense the seriousness of the moments; they abandoned their normal romps through the house during this somber time. And then it happened ... four or five hours before Jay took his last breath, the three dogs slowly and uncharacteristically walked into Jay's room in a single file, jumped onto the bed one at a time, and surrounded Jay. Together they simply lay by his side for approximately thirty minutes. Then, as suddenly as they came, they each got up and walked single file out of the room, never to enter the room again. They had said their good-byes, and they seemed to understand it was the end.

Conan was never the same after Jay died. He had clearly been Jay's dog. Before Jay's death, he would playfully nip Mary in the butt (Jay and Conan seemed to think this was funny), but this suddenly stopped the moment Jay died. Mary laughed when she told me that she secretly hoped that Jay had told Conan to be nicer to her now that the dog was going to have to depend on her once Jay was gone. Regardless of if this conversation occurred, Conan seemed to understand he was now Mary's dog.

The weeks that followed Jay's death were profoundly difficult for Mary. Her world had ended. This was the unexpected chapter in the story that was her life. Her story was supposed to end with happily ever after, and she now had no idea how to cope. As she sat in her chair in her grief, the dogs all came and sat beside her as if to comfort her. They seemed to know to just be, and all the normal mischievous behaviors subsided as if a dark cloud had consumed their home. And then, about three or four weeks after Jay's death, the dogs decided that was enough of the moping around. Conan found a pillow to destroy, blankets began to be used as tug toys, and the dogs collectively signaled it was time to get out of the house. Unable to ignore the escalating mayhem, Mary gathered the pups and began what would turn out to be a daily ritual of going to a nearby seventy-five-acre dog park. Watching her beloved pets romp in the fresh air, playing with the other park goers, began to heal her soul. Conan, Gizmo, and Sketch slowly reminded her that life goes on. It was hard not to smile at the canine antics of the dog park, and soon she was engaging in social banter with other dog owners. She remembered the bereavement classes offered by the hospice, and after attending them she began to emerge from the depths of sorrow.

Then Mary remembered the tiny westie and the joy the little pup brought to those he visited. She began to search online to learn more about the Delta Society and what it would take to get Conan registered as a therapy dog. Eager to make a difference for others, Conan and Mary took the test. Conan skillfully demonstrated his love for people as he eagerly greeted each person and wagged his tail in happy anticipation. Unfortunately, he also demonstrated his more stubborn side, refusing to sit on command at the crucial time. He failed the test. Mary was devastated, thinking, "I can't even do this!" She decided to retake the test with Sketch, only to witness Sketch obsessively focus on a toy that he was suppose to ignore. To Mary's disappointment, Sketch was only interested in the toys and in Mary, and showed little interest in interacting with others. He, too, failed.

Discouraged, Mary gave up on visiting with her dogs, and instead put her energies into helping a friend with rescue work. Then she received an e-mail from her friend with a picture of a liver and white ticked German wirehaired pointer. Her friend was asking if she knew anyone who would take the forty-five-pound, ten-year-old dog who would soon be euthanized if a suitable home was not found. The dog had been rescued from a home several states away. She had been chained outside after her owner had become overwhelmed with the responsibilities of caring for her three children, five dogs, and her own disability. There was no way she could care for everyone after her partner abandoned her, and the dogs were the first to go. The dog's eyes were soft and sweet as she stared at Mary from the picture. Mary immediately fell in love with the dog, but was reluctant to take her. Her last German wirehair pointer had come down with the very rare but serious Canine Rage Syndrome. The dog abruptly lunged from a deep sleep at Mary at two o'clock one morning. Had Mary not already been awake and somewhat alert, she most likely would not have been able to successfully fend off the dog until Jay could come to her rescue. The dog was then utterly confused, disoriented, and unaware of his actions after the attack. After extensive research into the uncommon condition, they decided they could no longer safely keep their beloved pet. It was heartbreaking for Mary, and although she understood how rare this medical condition is, she was apprehensive. She was not yet ready to open up her heart to yet another potential loss. But despite her fears, she decided to give it a shot.

Mary packed up her van and drove across state lines to pick up the pup. When she arrived at the designated truck stop, she was initially taken back by the crowd. Forty-some dogs had arrived, and adults and children intermingled with the dogs in a chaotic scene. And then, in the midst of it all, was the beautiful face from the picture. Mary knelt down to meet her, and the dog happily licked Mary's face in greeting and wagged her tail, seeming unfazed by the noise and disarray around them. Mary knew that very minute that this dog was hers. She named her Annie, and Annie marked the beginning of a new and joyous chapter for Mary.

Annie was a quick study. Although she had never been housebroken, she quickly learned from Mary's promptings and the disgusted looks from her canine housemates that relieving herself indoors was unacceptable. Within three days, she had that task mastered. Gizmo immediately assumed his typical role of ensuring that any newcomer toed the line, and he soon had Annie under his paw as well. Within twenty-four hours, Annie was seamlessly integrated into the family. Her mellow disposition was endearing and had a way of calming Mary's heart. When Mary and Annie began obedience classes, Mary was painfully aware that Annie had had a difficult life. Although Annie did not show any overt signs of past trauma, someone had most likely abused her, and Mary wanted to make sure that only empowering training techniques were used. After working together for six months, Mary and Annie took the Delta Society Pet Partners test, and to Mary's delight, they passed. Annie was a natural.

With Mary by her side, she visited in assisted living homes and worked in various medical settings. As we sat for our interview in the busy corridor of one of the assisted living homes, it was wonderful to witness Annie's natural talents as elderly residents stopped to visit with her. One gentleman wheeled by in his wheelchair in a white sailor's cap. "Look, Annie! There's the Admiral!" Mary exclaimed. Annie gave a doggy smile in recognition as she stood and made her way over for a visit. A warm smile spread across the kind man's face as he reached a shaky hand out to pet Annie's head. "I don't have any cookies for you today, Annie," he said; clearly wishing he had a treat for his beloved friend. Annie didn't seem to mind as she enjoyed the visit. As the visit came to an end, the gentleman said in a loving tone, "If I had a ranch, I'd have you, Annie." And with that he slowly wheeled his way toward the dining hall for dinner. Just a few minutes, but the short visit had made his day. The Admiral was just one of many who stopped for a visit during our time together. Staff and patients alike showed their love of Annie as they stopped for a quick snuggle.

Through their work together, Annie opened doors that Mary had been previously unable to open. Together they meet all types of wonderful people, and Mary now loves learning and becoming involved with different activities and projects. Annie has taught Mary how to approach people and how to find needed camaraderie. Mary confided that she had always depended on others to help her with that. Now with Annie by her side, she is able to move out of her comfort zone into a world she never knew existed.

Over the initial months that Mary and Annie worked together, Mary soon discovered that her greatest joy was working with those who had suffered from a stroke. She understood firsthand the frustration and pain that family members experience as they watch their loved ones struggle to find a word or to express themselves. She understood that the anger and outbursts are part of the aftermath of stroke and should not be taken personally. She was now ready to give back and find a way to help those who still had an opportunity to experience life after a stroke. Patients who struggled to hold a bar of soap soon found it helpful to hold Annie's brush (a similar size and shape) and practice their dexterity by brushing Annie's smooth coat. Mary patiently worked with those they visited through stories and conversation to help them formulate and express their thoughts. Annie also found a role in assisting wobbly patients as they practiced balance, walking beside her and using her for support as Mary guided the way. Mary soon learned that she and Annie could make a difference for these patients. With time, Mary returned to the very hospital where her beloved Jay had received care during those painful and trying months. It was the most painful place to visit. But, as Mary told me, she needed to do it to heal her soul and move on. Although Mary's life story did not follow the outline she had once prepared, and her dreams of living happily ever after seemed forever shattered, she now realized that a happy ending might somehow still be possible. Through their work together, Annie brought Mary full circle as she found the strength to close one chapter. As a result she is finally able to fully embrace the chapters yet to come.

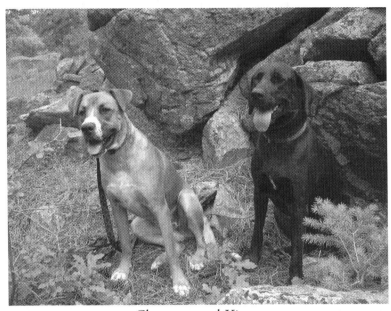

Cheyenne and Kiowa
*Photo by Sandra Owen*

# Chapter Thirteen
# Cheyenne and Kiowa

*The purpose of life is a life of purpose.*

—Robert Byrne

Some people believe in fate; others, in destiny. Still others believe that everything happens for a reason and by design. There are countless explanations for why each and every twist and turn of our lives occur. Living on this tiny planet requires a quest for meaning or understanding as our lives take unexpected paths. Despite each person's individual beliefs or ways of finding meaning, each of us is challenged to find our gifts and talents and to determine what we can do to fill the time that is our lives. Even when we think we have found our purpose in this world, how can we really be sure? It is often when we think we have found the answers that life throws us yet another curve ball, and we have to begin the searching all over again.

As I met all of the individuals and therapy dogs over the course of this year and heard each and every story, I noticed one thread they had in common. All were devoted dog lovers. Although for many, the dog was their first therapy dog, most had had dogs in childhood, and all had had dogs before beginning to work with their therapy dogs. All were self-professed dog lovers and already were well aware of the power of the human-animal bond. This was not an area that any of the people I interviewed ever questioned. I had come to expect that this pattern would continue, since clearly only a dog lover would devote the amount of time required to properly train and handle a therapy dog. True to life's patterns, just when I became comfortable and expected it to continue ... it changed.

After multiple e-mails to schedule a time to meet, I arrived at the urban medical center to meet Sandie and her therapy dog, Cheyenne. When I arrived, Cheyenne was happily napping under the information desk—to the delight of the volunteer—and she quickly said her good-byes as only a canine can do. Sandie led us back to a quiet conference room to chat. Those around us smiled at Cheyenne as we made our way through the maze of offices. Cheyenne (a beautiful boxer mix) watched attentively through the open doorway as we settled in and Sandie began to tell her story.

It was a hot August day in 2003 when Sandie, her husband, and her two grade-school-aged children were driving across Kansas, heading home from a family vacation. As they passed a roadside sign that indicated that they were nearing the Santa Fe Trail, they debated if they should stop and explore the point of interest. Deciding that the educational stop might be just what the family needed, they pulled into the parking lot and stretched their legs. The parking lot was deserted aside from an elderly man and two thin and disheveled dogs sitting near him. Thinking they must be the man's pets, they glanced at the man for permission to pet the animals as the dogs came near to visit. The man smiled, and the family petted and visited with the boxer mix and black lab. As the family walked along the trail and read the informational signs, the dogs stayed in close proximity. They chased the occasional rabbit, but quickly returned to stay within sight of the family. When it was time to leave, Sandie called to the man to please retrieve his dogs. To her surprise, he said they weren't his! With no one else in sight, to whom could these dogs belong? With concern rising, Sandie and her husband, Jeff, consulted to devise a plan. After a brief conversation, Sandie turned to discuss it further with the elderly man, only to realize that he had vanished and they were now alone with these two abandoned creatures.

Sandie knew that the dogs were depending on them and she felt a sense of obligation. However, Jeff did not feel as altruistic, and quickly reminded her that they did not have the time or resources to care for two strays. He went on to remind her that their two cats were not likely to be enthusiastic about an impromptu interspecies adoption. Despite Jeff's logic, Sandie's and her children's pleading wore him down, and it was agreed that the dogs could come along, but only until they could find them suitable assistance in town. So Jeff and Sandie put the dogs in the van, and the family headed back to Dodge City to look for help.

Despite their best efforts, help was not to be found. The veterinarian's office and the Humane Society were closed, and the police department was not willing to help yet another unwanted dog dumped along the highway. Coming to terms with the reality that these two dogs were going to be with the family for some time, they stopped at Wal-Mart for some basic pet supplies. When they offered their new travel mates some nourishment, however, the dogs refused to eat. Only later did the dogs show some interest in eating some French fries when the family pulled into a fast food restaurant. It was the only one they could enjoy now that the hot summer sun made it necessary to keep the dogs cool. Giving up being able to leave the car to enjoy a sit-down meal was a small price to pay for doing a good deed, Sandie concluded. Aside from one short-lived hopeful moment when the manager at Sonic thought he might know who owned the two dogs, the family gave up hope of finding the dogs' owner while they were on the road. They settled in for the five-hour ride back home, and began to pick out names for the pups— Cheyenne for the boxer mix, and Kiowa for the black lab.

Once the family arrived home, the cats confirmed Jeff's suspicions and made it known that they did not approve of the new houseguests. After Internet searches for possible matches to ads for lost dogs turned up nothing, Sandie quickly whisked the dogs to the local veterinarian for full workups. They were in bad shape; ticks, tapeworms, and mange were just a few of the initial problems. In addition, Cheyenne had apparently been hit by a car and needed embedded debris removed from her skin. The vet guesstimated the dogs' ages to be approximately ten months (as the pups became healthier, the vet later modified that guess to six months) and likely from the same litter. After she provided all the needed inoculations and medication, the vet sent them on their way with words of advice for Sandie. Sandie had never owned a dog before, and didn't know much about how to care for or understand dogs. While she did like dogs, she had always been a cat person, and this was a new experience. Eager to learn, Sandie signed herself and the pups up for obedience classes. She ran a tight household, and was determined to make her new canine houseguests tow the line.

Cheyenne, Kiowa, and Sandie were good studies. Not only did Cheyenne and Kiowa pass their obedience classes, they were the only dogs in their class to also pass their American Kennel Club Canine Good Citizen test. Sandie absorbed all she could, and she now was adept in canine culture and was deeply in love with both girls. (Need I mention that Jeff had now agreed to allow the family to keep both dogs?) They were indeed a part of the family; even the cats conceded the fight. Believing that the pups were destined for more, Sandie contacted her veterinarian once again to ask for ideas, and it was then that the veterinarian told Sandie about therapy dog work. Sandie was incensed! How could she ever suggest that she give up these dogs after all that they had been through! She had fallen in love with these animals, and would not ever consider giving them away! After the veterinarian patiently clarified that therapy dogs are not the same as service dogs and that therapy dogs are kept and handled by their owners, Sandie gathered herself to listen to the idea. When she learned about the Delta Society and the resultant possibilities, it sounded perfect.

Having a nurse for a mother, Sandie had always dreamed of being a hospital volunteer, and the idea of volunteering with her beloved pets was just what she needed. After researching available testing sites, Sandie pulled into the parking lot with her dogs for the exam. She and Kiowa tested first, but she was horrified to discover she could hear Cheyenne's cries of displeasure from the car where she had left her. Cheyenne hated being left alone, and to Sandie's dismay, she was making her feelings loudly known. After passing the test with Kiowa, she was sure that Cheyenne had already failed (potential therapy dogs are tested on all behaviors they exhibit while on the property, even when not being formally tested). Sure that the evaluator was just being polite by asking Sandie to bring Cheyenne in for the formal test, she complied. She was thrilled to learn that Cheyenne passed the exam as well.

And so began a new chapter for Sandie, Cheyenne, and Kiowa. They began regularly visiting at a local medical center, and Sandie soon became the team lead for the visiting pet partners at the medical center. Before long she discovered that her full-time work as assistant director at an after-school child care center was getting in the way of the time she wanted to spend volunteering. She had found her purpose in life. Seeing the joy that his wife was getting from her volunteer work, Jeff agreed they could survive without the extra income; freeing her up to spend her time in the environment she loved.

It was the perfect environment for them, and they were instant hits. Since the hospital only allowed one dog to visit each floor per day, each dog had her own day. Cheyenne and Kiowa each seemed to sense that it was all about her on her special day. As they settled into their routine, Sandie soon learned how unique each dog is in how she visits and approaches her job. Cheyenne prefers to sit in a chair beside her patients' bed. She calmly waits while Sandie gently slides the chair close to the bed, and then sits quietly enjoying the patient's touch. In one room, Sandie discovered one of Cheyenne's many quirks; she loves to watch herself in the mirror. In this particular room, the mirror is directly across from where Cheyenne sits on her chair to visit, and nothing will distract her from admiring herself in the mirror. Sandie covers for Cheyenne by explaining that she is trained not to lick IV sites, so she often looks away while being petted. However, patients now find it comical that Cheyenne can not be dissuaded from admiring herself in the mirror.

Cheyenne is a dog on the move. She gets antsy being in one place too long. Even during my interview, she began to vocalize quietly to let us know that we might have more fun in the hallway. Kiowa is more of a snuggler. She has a calming nature, and finds a way to lie on her chair beside the patient and gently put her head and paws close to the patient to give a small-dog feel. She has a very special way of making each person feel as though he or she is the only person in Kiowa's world, as if there is no place else the dog would rather be.

As Sandie spoke about her work with her beloved pets, she laughed as she explained how her "girls" are able to win the hearts even of cat lovers. One day at the hospital she offered a visit with Cheyenne only to be told by a patient, "No thanks, I'm more of a cat person."

Sandie quickly replied, "Oh, Cheyenne's a cat person, too!" She retrieved a picture of Cheyenne curled up with the family cat. Soon the patient was smiling and enjoying a visit with her new canine friend.

As my questions turned to explore how working with Cheyenne and Kiowa had changed Sandie, she smiled and quickly referred to a small piece of paper. "I've been thinking a lot about that," she said. Her love for her pups was clearly evident as she joked about never realizing before how much she needs an escort to go from room to room in her home (yes, even to the bathroom), how comfortable sitting on the floor watching television could be with a dog on each side, or how wonderful it feels to have a warm friend sleep on her feet. She has discovered all the many luxuries in life that all of the rest of us dog lovers have always known.

She then told me how adopting these two stray dogs on that hot summer day has transformed her as a human being. She is now a much better listener ("although not always at home," she jokes) and is much less judgmental of those whom she hears. She tells me how much her patients just need someone who will listen to them, someone who won't stick them with a needle or give them a pill. She went on to tell me how visiting prisoners in the hospital has changed her. She used to be nervous around them and think they were just getting what they deserved, but has since learned that despite being chained to the bed for some crime, they, too, deserve some compassion and "warm fuzzy time." She is now able to table her emotions and judgments to be present with those she visits. In doing so, she has found true joy. She has found that in giving, she only wants to give more.

She soon discovered that there was something more that she needed to be doing in this life; she had a greater purpose. Through adopting her two pups and raising them to help others, she discovered that she has a gift for nurturing and fostering those in need. This opened up a door for Sandie, and she is now taking classes to learn to be a foster parent for babies for the local child protective services. Through working with her therapy dogs, she learned the skills to set aside her judgment and help others. It is these skills that will be instrumental in her success in showing empathy and in helping to care for another mother's child in a time in need.

Cheyenne and Kiowa have won the hearts of an entire cat family. Laughter over Cheyenne's quirks is now commonplace, and even the strict Jeff has been known to allow a dog on the couch from time to time. The kids love to sit with the dogs in the van and they now depend on their canine buddies to wake them in the mornings. And, because of Cheyenne and Kiowa, a baby's cry will soon be heard throughout the home, reminding all of the power of giving. Sandie now believes that she was meant to find Cheyenne and Kiowa along the Santa Fe Trail on that hot summer day. It was not an accident. They were waiting just for her. Although her husband now jokes that they can never go on a road trip again (the souvenirs are just too expensive!), she knows that it was meant to be. Through her "puppy girls" she has found her purpose, and she knows how lucky she is to be one of the few who has found her mission in this world.

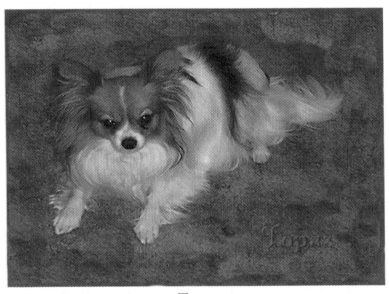

Topaz
*Photo by Teresa Knisley*

# Chapter Fourteen
# Topaz

*Acquiring a dog may be the*
*only opportunity a human ever*
*has to choose a relative.*

— Mordecai Siegal

In America we live in a very materialistic society. Media messages tell consumers that we should purchase the latest car, fashion, or gadget because we are "worth it" or because we "deserve it." When I work with discouraged parents of wayward adolescents, they are frequently dismayed at the parenting adage that adolescents should earn extras as a way of learning how to be responsible adults, and they are even more surprised to learn that designer clothing, dining out, and entertainment could possibly be considered extras. These one-time luxuries are commonly considered to be essentials in today's culture. Many of my clients are relatively poor. Housing and employment are common problems with which they struggle, yet despite their socioeconomic status, they frequently have the latest cell phone and cable television. We live in a society of excess, with little thought given to how one will pay for all these items that we all "deserve."

Growing up, money was rather tight. My mother chose to stay home when we were young, and my father worked long hours and often traveled around the country in his job as an auditor. Meals were made from scratch, and pasta, potatoes, and beans were frequent menu items. My mother made many of our clothes, and we were taught to value what we had; should something break, we knew it most likely would not be replaced. It was difficult going to school and seeing my classmates wearing the latest fashions, while I was wearing my sister's or cousin's hand-me-downs from the previous decade. This was when I first learned how cruel children could be to those who look different. I didn't understand at the time why I could not have the latest designer tennis shoes or jeans. Somehow I thought I would fit in better if I only could dress like everyone else. My parents did their best, and in looking back I now appreciate the lessons I learned from those difficult years. As an adult, I often hear friends and colleagues make mention of the mounting stress and debt resulting from getting the latest gadget, while simultaneously making reference to the fact that they had worked hard and therefore deserved the cherished item. While I am not immune to enjoying the occasional creature comfort, somewhere along the road I began to understand that my self worth was not connected to having the latest gadget, and that often the best reward is not associated with a material object.

I have been described by friends and colleagues as a type of social rebel. When there is a mainstream of thought, I most likely disagree with it. Maybe that is one of the reasons I was attracted to the advocacy nature of the field of social work. I can also be rather black and white in my thought process, resulting in me thinking through ideas to the ridiculous level to ensure they remain logical from all angles. All of this has resulted in me adopting what I have come to term the "dumb luck" theory of life in order to make sense of how someone in America can be a millionaire and yet be miserable and someone in a mud hut on the other side of the world can be so happy. It has nothing to do with what we deserve. It is about what we do with what we have. We have all been dealt a different set of cards. We aren't dealt these cards according to what we deserve, for we are all equal on that level. Rather, they are given to us in a random fashion, making some wealthy, some poor, some healthy, and some with illness. None deserves more than the other, and yet some receive more by the luck of the draw. Success is ultimately measured by how we play our hand. But there are things each of us can do to better our odds of winning despite the cards we were initially dealt. We are not helpless victims, doomed to accept our predetermined fate. Our dear animal friends teach us this important lesson as they demonstrate that happiness is not connected to material possessions or health, but to a love of life and a deep appreciation of who is in our lives. This is the story of Topaz.

Teresa had a difficult start in life. Her mother married at the tender age of fifteen, and Teresa was born just one year later. Raising children is difficult enough, but it is even more challenging when the parents are only adolescents themselves. Teresa became very close to her father as a child; she was a daddy's girl by most definitions. Unfortunately, the unintended consequence was jealousy from her mother and a strained relationship that continued throughout her life. Her mother's criticism left her questioning herself and avoiding new situations. Teresa made the most of it, but would not describe her family as supportive or close. She was dealt a difficult hand of cards. Always wanting to help others, she became a nurses' aide and later taught preschool when she left home.

Then in 1997, her knee began to swell and cause her tremendous pain. After consulting with several doctors, she determined that she was suffering from an abscess. Relieved to have finally been given a diagnosis, she was then disappointed to learn that the doctors did not think it required surgery, even though she was beginning to have difficulty walking. Undeterred, she found another doctor who was willing to do exploratory surgery to discover what was causing such discomfort. The day before the surgery was scheduled, she misstepped, injuring her knee even more so that she required emergency surgery. Teresa emerged from the surgery to learn that she had had a cyst the size of a baseball in her knee; it had burst, destroying parts of her knee cap, and the doctors had had to pack it with cadaver bone in order to repair it. Since she was unable to stand for long periods of time, it was difficult for her to work. Although she requested schedule changes and other accommodations that would allow her to continue working, it became too arduous, and she eventually decided it was better for everyone if she quit.

Teresa's knee made it impossible for her to hold a full-time job, but she still longed to help others. She knew herself well. She was an introvert, and without external obligations she would most likely stay at home watching television, listening to music, or playing computer games. Eager to fill her time, she began to volunteer at local health fairs and other charitable events. These events became social avenues, a way that she could still contribute to society despite her disability. Then a friend suggested that Teresa look into volunteering with her dogs as a way to combine her love of dogs and her volunteer work. It seemed like the ideal solution. Teresa had always loved dogs. When she was younger she and her brother had bred and raised powder-puff Chinese cresteds. Her brother stopped, but her love for the breed continued, and she began helping local rescues by fostering the little pups. They were the perfect size, less than fifteen pounds. She ended up adopting two adorable pups, Inky and Lilly. At the ripe old age of seventeen and a half, the day came for Inky to pass. Missing her little friend, Lilly began to get depressed, and Teresa knew it was time to find another dog to join their family. Knowing that the perfect dog would be of similar size, she began to research shih tzu, Maltese, and papillon pups, hoping to find the ideal temperament. This would be the first dog she raised from a puppy, and she worked hard to ensure the dog was perfect. Before finalizing her decision, she agreed to foster two papillons to get a sense of their true personality and temperament. This trial run was just what she needed to finally settle upon a breeder in South Carolina, and her little five-month-old papillon was soon in transit to the local airport. Intent that the transition go well, she had followed the breeder's instructions to mail a shirt she had worn to be placed in her puppy's crate to allow the dog to become familiar with her scent. In addition, she had brainstormed many names for her new little friend, but it wasn't until the moment she opened the crate and saw the sun's rays playfully dance upon the sable and white colored three-pound pup that she knew the perfect name. There in the sun she could see an unmistakable red tint. "Topaz," she said happily, as she held the pup close.

Topaz and Teresa were close from the start. Maybe it was the T-shirt she had sent ahead—at least that is how Teresa explains it. Over the next year, Teresa patiently worked to socialize her tiny friend and teach her basic manners. They even tried agility class only to learn that it was not for Topaz. She was a quiet dog who preferred to snuggle. Other than the occasional outburst over a pesky squirrel taunting her outside the living room window, she was content to sleep comfortably next to Teresa. When Topaz turned one year old, Teresa decided it was time to follow up on the leads she had found earlier to become a therapy dog team. She signed up for the handler's course, but she and Topaz then failed the exam. Topaz was not comfortable walking through a crowd, and definitely did not enjoy being placed on a stranger's lap for petting (both required elements of the test). Determined to help her little friend through these challenging parts, Teresa signed up for additional classes at the local pet store and solicited help from strangers to help her overcome Topaz's apprehension of sitting on strangers' laps. And then ... only a few months later, they passed the exam. In addition to taking the standard therapy dog exam, Teresa decided to complete the Reading Education Assistance Dog (R.E.A.D.) course that would allow them to work in schools and libraries. Although she wasn't really sure how Topaz would do around children, she thought it might be a worthwhile credential.

Now qualified to visit, Teresa began to search for the perfect location. Although she entertained the idea of visiting in hospitals, she worried that she would be unable to navigate the labyrinth of long hallways and corridors with her limited mobility. When the idea of visiting schools was suggested, she hesitantly agreed, still uncertain how Topaz would feel about working with children. The school was close to Teresa's home, and this added convenience increased its appeal. On the first day at the elementary school, Teresa could feel Topaz's apprehension as they entered the building. Topaz was not her typical fun-loving self, and Teresa had to coax her through the doors. But when Teresa thought to pick up her little partner, Topaz suddenly regained her confidence and showed Teresa that she could happily work in such a setting. Soon they were working with the children each week as Topaz attentively listened to the students reading books of assorted topics.

It was both a challenging and wonderful first year. Teresa had assisted Topaz in conquering her fears, and the shy duo were soon loved by the students and teachers. However, unbeknownst to those around her, Teresa was struggling with continued medical problems. She would suddenly experience hot flashes (similar to those experienced after heavy exercise), lightheadedness, stomach pain, and bouts of vomiting. Visits to her doctor revealed nothing significant, and she was repeatedly told it was most likely the onset of menopause or the flu. Frustrated at her continued symptoms with no apparent cause, she went about her daily routine. She believed that something was wrong, but she could not convince a doctor to do further investigation. Then one day, she suffered a heart attack. This was by far the most terrifying time in Teresa's life. She was rushed to the hospital, and doctors decided the best treatment was a coronary artery bypass graft (or shunt), during which they took a vessel from another part of her body and grafted it onto her coronary arteries in two places to provide alternative routes for the blood flow. During this hospital stay, they determined that Teresa's previous symptoms were most likely related to earlier heart damage, and that she was also suffering from a defective mitral valve.

Once released from the hospital she returned home. Her beloved pups were her primary family, and being with Lilly and

Topaz helped her through the difficult times. They depended on each other, and the little pups knew when something was wrong. On one occasion, Teresa stood up from the couch only to discover that she was too weak to walk. She then toppled onto the floor, landing on her shoulder. Topaz agilely moved out of the way to avoid the falling woman. She then turned back to Teresa and began to lick her face, doing her best to comfort her. Knowing she was injured from the fall, Teresa managed to call her mother for assistance. She had torn her rotator cuff, which resulted in additional surgery. Through it all, Teresa became even closer to Lilly and Topaz. They were the ones who were there for her each day. They made her smile during the toughest of times, and forced her to get up and care for them when she would rather stay in bed and fall prey to her depression. Her neighbors kept a close eye out for Teresa, watching to ensure the dogs were let out back on occasion each day as a sign that all was well within the residence.

With time, Teresa began to recover from the heart attack and her shoulder surgery. She slowly returned to her volunteer work at the nearby elementary school and began to once again foster dogs in need. One such dog was Fonzy, a little papillon who was rescued after becoming overly rambunctious with his owner's daughter. Fonzy had come from a puppy mill and needed more than this young family could offer. Without the proper training and attention, Fonzy began to show behavior problems that just could not be tolerated around young children. Teresa described Fonzy as a "border collie in disguise." He loved to chase anything that moved, and could not be fed with the other dogs. Left unattended he was soon rummaging through the garbage, and frequent neighborhood walks were necessary to minimize the chaos. Soon she was walking Lilly, Topaz, and Fonzy several times each day; keeping a watchful eye to ensure that Topaz didn't wander underfoot. Teresa also found that Fonzy did best when she was teaching him tricks to keep his brain occupied and out of trouble, so soon she had him crawling, sitting up, winking, and fetching on command. For some reason she only succeeded in getting Fonzy to fetch three consecutive times; the fourth time he decided that retrieving the object was up to Teresa. Before long, Teresa was in love with Fonzy, and she decided to adopt him as well. His quirks and silly disposition were just too endearing to pass up.

Speaking with Teresa by phone gave me a wonderful picture of Teresa and her three little pups, but I wanted to meet Topaz to truly get a sense of this little pup in action. A few weeks later, I sat in my car in the elementary school parking lot watching the children on the playground. I was careful to keep an eye out for Topaz; knowing that Teresa tired easily and not wanting her to wait on my behalf. And then, out of the corner of my eye, I saw a tiny white and brown dog running around her owner as they stood outside the school. I gathered my things and hurried over, only to see them disappear into the school before I could catch them. Once in the school, I looked down each hallway, eager to locate them. Then to my left, I saw them in the school office. Teresa held Topaz's leash at shoulder height to keep it from getting in the tiny dog's way as she scurried around the room visiting the office staff. Big smiles were on the staff members' faces as they bent down to greet their little friend.

Teresa mentioned that Lilly was very sick. The ten-year-old dog had stopped eating several days ago, and Teresa had come to terms that this was most likely the end for her dear older dog. Lilly had suffered from epilepsy for most of her life, and Teresa had managed to decrease the symptoms by controlling her diet. She told me that she had decided to allow Lilly to go if it was her time rather than seeking heroic medical efforts, given her chronic condition and old age. She had traveled that medical path with previous dogs, she told me, but it was time to just let go. I could only imagine how difficult it must be for Teresa, and I was silently amazed she had not canceled her volunteer work that day.

Then I realized what a blessing this work is for her. It is her way of escaping the medical woes and worries that encompass the rest of her life. As we said our good-byes to the office staff and started toward the door, I was immediately struck by how different it is to walk beside a tiny dog who weighs in the teens compared to my eighty pound collie. Teresa was ever- hypervigilant of where Topaz was as we traveled through the hallway, but the dog skill-fully demonstrated her comfort and ease as children stopped us in the hallway for a quick visit. The children's affect immediately changed when they saw Topaz, and joyful squeals abounded as they came over to pet her soft fur.

Once at the classroom, Teresa momentarily disappeared into the dark room as she gathered an additional chair and set it beside a desk just outside the second grade classroom doorway and up against the brightly painted yellow hallway wall. She then reached into her tote bag to retrieve a purple fleece blanket decorated with colorful patterns of butterflies and ladybugs, which she care-fully spread across the desktop. Children quickly gathered, and happy chatter filled the halls as Teresa gently lifted Topaz onto the blanket-covered desk. She arranged a small water dish (barely a swallow for my big dogs), a button decorated with Topaz's pic-ture, an array of colorful pencils, a stack of photographs of Topaz and assorted children, and a large self-inking rubber stamp. She carefully sorted an array of children's books into a box that she set on the floor nearby. All the while, children came up to Topaz to enjoy a quick snuggle. Once settled, Teresa kindly instructed the children to ask the teacher who would be first; she handed one of the children the "Topaz button" to indicate who would be first to read that day. Throughout the preparation ritual, Topaz sat proudly on her purple blanket enjoying the attention. On oc-casion, Teresa dabbed her finger into the water bowl and tapped the water onto Topaz's nose and tongue. "She gets so hot," Teresa explained. She told me this would be the last week for the school year. "It just gets too hot for both of us."

A Hispanic child eagerly made herself comfortable in the chair, scooted the chair up to the desk, and handed the Topaz button back to Teresa. She opened her book about sharks and began to read. Not the warm fuzzy topic I would have expected from a girl her age, but Topaz didn't seem fazed as the child read about the sharp teeth and other carnivore characteristics of this marine creature. As she read, the child's attention was not deterred despite children and adults occasionally walking down the hallway and reacting in happy surprise at seeing Topaz upon her perch. Once the girl was finished reading, Teresa invited her to look through the photographs to find the picture of her posing with Topaz. The child smiled in recognition as she took a picture. She then selected a pencil and a book from the stack on the floor. Once she had selected her treasures, Teresa showed her how to have Topaz "sign" the book by using the personalized rubber stamp of Topaz's paw print. In a farewell gesture, the girl gave Topaz a parting pat and disappeared into the classroom as another child quickly took her place in the chair; eager to read the story about a cat to Topaz.

After reading with several children, Teresa declared that their time was over and packed away her treasures for another day. She then lifted little Topaz and carried her down the hallway. Topaz gave her little doggy smile and made an endearing grunting sound as she relaxed into Teresa's arms. "That's her purring sound that she makes when she is happy," Teresa explained. Teresa tires quite easily, and she can only listen to a few children for a half hour. "We will be back next year," she promised.

In witnessing those hallway interactions that day, it became clear the difference Topaz makes for Teresa. Topaz is her motivation to get out of the house, and these visits give Teresa joy in helping others. In order to solicit donations of gifts for the children, she must contact others and talk about her work. Teresa may not have been dealt the most coveted hand of cards. Each day, medical problems and fears about what lies ahead plague her. But her story is a poignant reminder that it is not the cards we have been dealt that matter most in this world, but the way we play our hand.

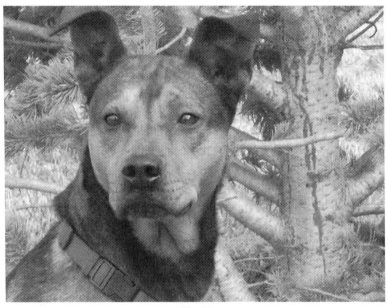

Katie
*Photo by Kathie Young*

# Chapter Fifteen
# Katie

*Children and dogs are as*
*necessary to the welfare of the*
*country as Wall Street and the*
*railroads.*

—Harry S. Truman

There is something both deeply personal and powerful about a well-written story. However, when one gives only the facts of the matter, the story can be rather mechanical and insipid. While the words may be accurate, the resulting tale is devoid of life and soul. I love to read. However, I must confess that there are some books that just simply do not hold my attention. My bookshelves are littered with partially read tomes, with scraps of paper marking the spot at which my interest was officially lost. I've never taken the time to analyze what was different about the author's style so that it could not hold my focus, but it is instantly apparent to me when I crack the spine of a book that is destined to pull me into the story line and leave me wanting more. When I find such a book, I eagerly search for everything that author has written, knowing that I will truly enjoy each story told. One such author is Jon Katz.

I was introduced to Jon Katz's work during one of those fleeting interactions between dog owners. It was late one Friday afternoon, and I was attempting to sneak a peek through the venetian blinds that cover the window between the waiting area and the canine play yard at the doggie daycare Jasper sometimes attends. Jasper is an extremely active dog, and we have learned through trial and error that having a professional and a willing crew of playful canines exhaust our dog from time to time is a wise investment. I love to see Jasper playfully romp with his canine buddies as the daycare attendant does his best to get Jasper's attention to send him home. In addition, I had come to look forward to the days that this particular daycare attendant was working. He had long black hair pulled back into an unruly ponytail. His thin arms were covered with colorful tattoos, and his facial hair provided just the finishing touches to result in a young man who in many other circumstances I most likely would have feared. However, in this setting, he was simply the wonderfully friendly daycare attendant, Patrick. He clearly loved the dogs, and the dogs responded in kind. He provided detailed reports about Jasper's antics, and he seemed to genuinely enjoy giving me the blow-by-blow on Jasper's day. Today was no exception. Patrick smiled as he handed me Jasper's leash and told me how tired he was due to the crazy antics of the "three psychotic musketeers" (it did not surprise me that my own little Jasper was one of these exhausting pups). He went on to tell me that Jasper, another rough coat collie, and a border collie had spent the day herding the other twenty-four dogs into calculated subgroups only to move them once again into different configurations. He laughed as he said that the other dogs didn't seem to mind; seemingly oblivious as to the reasons behind this odd running game the herding dogs had devised. Jasper had merely slowed to take the mandatory break around noon, only to instigate his two buddies in playing another round once Patrick and the other attendant released the dogs to play again that afternoon. "That dog doesn't stop!" Patrick said as I turned to leave. Then he asked in a parting thought if I had ever read the book, *A Dog Year*, by Jon Katz (2003); saying that Jasper reminded him of the unruly border collie that was the book's main character. Something about the twinkle in Patrick's eye enticed me into buying the book.

As I settled into a comfy wicker glider on the back deck, I was instantly hooked by the stories, and I laughed until I cried, enjoying every moment. There was something so poignant about the way the author interwove his personal thoughts with the story line that touched deep into my soul. It wasn't long before I had purchased all the books Katz had authored and was lost within the pages as my pups slept peacefully by my side. It was Katz who introduced me to the concept that if one wants to have a better-behaved dog, one has to be a better human. It was a concept that transformed me to my core and has changed my personal and professional life profoundly. His ability to speak to the reader on a personal level while telling a simple story is the hallmark of a gifted writer. Writing is often an avenue of personal expression, as the writers blend their own personal struggles and reflections into the stories told. And it was this genuine blending of personal vulnerability loosely veiled within the story that caught my interest as Anne told me about her beloved Katie.

On a sunny spring afternoon, I parked my car and walked up the steps of the old building where I was to meet Anne and her canine partner, Katie. The old brick building was constructed in 1902 as an orphanage, and now houses up to forty children and adolescents who are struggling with severe behavioral and mental health problems. The hallways were dark, and the carpet and furnishings showed their age as I followed echoing sounds in an effort to find Anne and Katie. On occasion a small group of well-mannered adolescents accompanied by a staff member passed me in the corridor, barely giving me a glace. The worn stairs creaked beneath their weight as the residents climbed them. Before long I heard the tattletale jingle of a dog's leash, and looked up to see a smiling silver-haired woman in her sixties and a sweet Rhodesian ridgeback mix coming toward me. After brief introductions, we made our way to a quiet room to visit. Here is the story she told.

Katie came into Anne's life by accident one spring day in 2003. Just three days earlier, Anne's nine-year-old husky mix, Kachina, had lost her fight with kidney disease and had left Anne heartbroken. Kachina had somehow survived an aggressive cancerous tumor on her nose, but she was unable to conquer her fight with kidney disease. So on this spring day, with the emptiness of the house too much to bear, Anne found herself walking alone with a heavy heart. There in the neighborhood park, she saw her friend, Jane, with not only her own two dogs, but a third on a long rope. When she stopped to chat, her friend's story came tumbling out. Jane works with feral cats, feeding and trapping them to take the creatures to the veterinarian for care. She had been working one of her feral cat colonies a few hours earlier when she saw a five- to eight-month-old pup running down the sidewalk. She could tell, even from a distance, that the dog did not have a collar or any identification tags. Concerned, she did her best to coax the young dog to her, only spooking the dog and making it sprint in the opposite direction. An animal lover at heart, Jane followed at a safe distance in hopes of gaining the dog's trust so she could bring the animal to safety. To her surprise, the dog ran onto the porch of a nearby home despite being seemingly frightened by the two residents loitering on the home's wide porch. Overcome by her love of animals, Jane began to berate the men for allowing their young dog to wander the streets unattended, only to be met with the callous reply, "Hey, she knows where she lives!" Taking a deep breath to control her growing frustration, she stayed and engaged in a conversation with the two men. She learned that the dog had been owned by one of the men's sister but that she had given the dog up. Just when Jane was turning to walk away to contemplate a different plan of attack, one of the men said, "Do you want her?" Startled by the impromptu offer, Jane quickly accepted and hurried away with the timid dog in tow before the men could change their minds. After a brief stop back home to invite her own dogs to join them, they continued to the neighborhood park where Jane could ponder her next steps.

Anne knew immediately that she wanted this dog, but when Jane made the official offer once they had returned to Jane's home, Anne also knew she was not ready. Not quite yet. She had always been a serial dog owner; having just one dog at a time. Now that Kachina was gone, she knew she would soon find another, but it seemed too soon; she still missed her little buddy deeply. The newly rescued dog playfully nipped at Anne's arms and legs as if to engage her as they visited, but she readily stopped when Anne informed her that this was not the way to a human's heart. Anne could tell how intelligent she was, and this further endeared the young pup to Anne. Then Jane devised a plan. What if Anne took the dog overnight and on weekends until she was ready to take her full time? It was the perfect solution. They soon settled on the name, Katie, and the scheduled visitation plan began. Anne dutifully brought Katie to Jane's house on her way to work, and then picked her up again on her way home. Katie had the best of both worlds. Jane was home most of the day caring for her young child, and Katie was able to accompany her on her regular trips to tend to the feral cats. She then enjoyed an evening of pampering with Anne. Katie could not have been happier. Three weeks later, Anne decided she was ready, and officially moved Katie to her forever home.

All of Anne's previous dogs were rescues. Her dog before Kachina was Dagny, a terrier mix. And, like many of us, Anne had slowly learned over the years about dog culture and what these creatures truly need for good physical and emotional health. When Anne adopted Dagny, it was a different time in American culture; dogs were viewed simply as animals and were seldom afforded the luxuries of the dogs of today. Anne had rescued this dear little pup when Anne was younger and much more active. She has since undergone two hip replacements, making her previous active lifestyle impossible with Katie. In those earlier years Anne placed a cardboard box and blanket on the covered back porch for Dagny when she was at work and the weather permitted. After discovering Dagny's ability to scale the back fence and escape, Anne devised a way to tie her on an ample leash in the backyard to keep her from escaping while still allowing her to enjoy the fresh air. They would then bicycle, hike, and enjoy all sorts of other outdoor activities together during Anne's leisure time. During one of these relished activities, Dagny took her last breath as she unwittingly stepped of a cliff during a hike. She was nine and a half years old, and she must have been becoming blind, deaf, or disoriented to have made such a misstep, surmised Anne. It was a loss that devastated Anne. Anne implemented the lessons learned when she adopted Kachina. Yet, even Kachina lived a life far different from Katie's. Anne purchased a well-insulated hand-constructed wooden dog house with a shingle roof for her canine friend to make her time outside enjoyable. Needless to say, Katie was not sleeping in a cardboard box on the back porch or tethered in the backyard. In fact, Katie would have nothing to do with the state-of-the-art dog house that Kachina had once enjoyed. Anne had since learned about the importance of good canine dental hygiene and other needs, and Katie enjoyed a pampered life indoors with Anne.

During the first week, Anne discovered one of Katie's quirks. She was incredibly anxious when left alone. On one occasion, Katie escaped from her crate, went out the doggie door, jumped the fence, and headed back to Jane's house. On other occasions, she chewed the mini blinds, tore the drapes, and got up onto the countertops. When left in her crate, she was just as anxious and destructive as she chewed up her blankets. Katie was an amazingly calm dog until there was any inkling that Anne was about to leave. Resigned to having to arrange for someone to stay with Katie while she worked, she began taking Katie to a family's home near her work in the hospital, or dropping her off at Jane's house when needed. Years later, during one final attempt to see if Katie could manage being alone, she left Katie at home while she went to the grocery store. She was gone no more than twenty minutes. When she turned the corner toward home, to her horror, she found Katie, hyperventilating, on the street corner in her neighborhood after she had escaped yet again. It was then that Anne finally decided she simply could not leave Katie alone. During cooler weather, she left Katie in the car as she ran errands, finding that Katie was somehow able to manage her anxiety during these short stints as long as she was safely in the vehicle. Katie would even come along to outdoor restaurants that would allow the dog to sit in the patio area. Anne resigned herself to the idea that this was a quirk she would have to accept.

During the few weeks after Katie's rescue, she had become very attached to Jane's family. Jane was with her continuously, and the transition to a new home proved difficult. Anne and Katie frequently saw Jane and her family in the neighborhood park, and Katie's plaintive cries and whimpers were common when the time came to part. Although it was heartbreaking for Anne, she was determined to help Katie through. She now loved this dog and couldn't imagine life without her. However, it wasn't just Katie who was having a difficult adjustment. Anne suffered from nagging fears that she was not doing a good enough job with Katie, fears that the previous owner would recognize Katie and want her back. Knowing that Katie was rescued less than a mile from her home, she would sometimes wonder if the person she saw on the street or at the neighborhood park was one of the men about whom Jane had spoken. Together Anne and Katie participated in obedience classes and other group activities, and slowly, they were able to set aside their difficult emotions and bond to each other.

So many times I have heard therapy dog handlers say that their dogs were perfect from the start; that the dog was such a natural that formal training was only a formality. While I have no reason to think these people are being untruthful, I am always relieved to hear about dogs like Katie since they are much more representative of the average dog. Katie was a dog with issues. In fact I have always found these more typical dogs to be the most inspirational and helpful during therapy dog workshops and classes, for they teach us the importance of being aware of whom our dogs are and taking the time to help them be the best dogs they can be. They teach us that dogs and humans can overcome adversity and obstacles with patience and by keeping our eyes on the goal. Of all the therapy dog stories I have heard, Katie is my favorite in this regard. Her path to becoming a therapy dog was not easy; it is a story of perseverance and persistence. Hers is the story of a dog that under most circumstances would have been simply a household pet.

Katie could best be described as a sweet dog with tremendous baggage. Even after she bonded with Anne she cowered, apprehensive of strangers, particularly large men or those with darker skin tones. Anne knew that Katie most likely had not been properly socialized, so she made tremendous effort to show her the world. As they took long walks in more secluded areas, Katie would frequently stop and cock her head in curiosity, as she tried to understand the sounds and the cars moving in the distance. On one of their weekend outings, Anne happened across an animal communicator working a booth at a local animal-themed affair at an area park. Eager to learn if this professional could give her some insight into Katie and her continued separation anxiety, she stopped. It was then that Anne first learned about therapy dogs, for the animal communicator suggested that Katie would be good at this activity. She also suggested agility as a way to solidify their bond. Although initially very surprised by this suggestion—Katie was still struggling with nervousness around strangers—Anne immediately was attracted to this idea. She knew she wanted to engage in some form of volunteer work, and with her retirement on the horizon, this might be just the thing.

And then almost by design, she saw a poster the very next day at the hospital at which she worked about the therapy dog program they were planning to start. Although the poster had most likely been there for quite some time, it wasn't until the thought had been planted that it caught her eye. She eagerly gathered information about the process, and explored the next steps. Anne then completed the handlers' course and scheduled the exam, only to cancel it when she realized she and Katie simply were not ready. But this became her goal—to volunteer with Katie. She found a local agility class, and this was something they both enjoyed until Anne was no longer able to keep up with her agile canine friend. She took the Canine Good Citizen exam through the American Kennel Club, but to her disappointment, they failed. Anne had not yet understood that they were not only testing Katie, but they were testing her ability to help her dog succeed. It was a difficult but necessary lesson. In addition, she located a trainer who was familiar with the therapy dog requirements to help her target some of Katie's problem areas. Together with the trainer, they began an intensive training program. The trainer made loud noises and rattled items as Anne and Katie walked in public settings, and they practiced visiting anyone who was willing.

Determined to reach her goal, Anne decided to join the therapy dog organization without her dog, and she faithfully attended the monthly meetings to take advantage of the support and information, even though she silently longed to have her canine companion by her side. Together she and Katie continued their training; ignoring a neutral dog and approaching strangers continued to be challenging. In retrospect, the process itself was a gift to Anne, for she gained a tremendous sense of accomplishment as she set specific goals and then worked with Katie to achieve them. For example, even after Katie had overcome her apprehension of most strangers, she continued to bark and be uncomfortable around one particular gentleman. He was a large man with a beard and long red hair tied back into a ponytail. Determined to help Katie overcome her fear, Anne arranged to meet the gentleman in a neighborhood park with the dog trainer, and helping Katie overcome this fear became the goal for the day. By the end of the session, Katie discovered that there was nothing to fear, and soon she was enjoying a snuggle with her new friend.

With time, she passed the Canine Good Citizen test, and then even the therapy dog exam. Anne could not have been prouder of Katie.

Anne is a nurse by profession. She completed her bachelor's degree in nursing and worked for several years to hone her skills before striking out to volunteer at a health department in a state far away from her family in Michigan. While she was initially taken aback by the ethnic diversity and presence of bars and other establishments that had not been common in her small hometown, she came to love her new state, and never returned to Michigan. As a single woman, she took full advantage of her freedoms, and accepted nursing jobs that allowed her to return to school on many occasions throughout her adult life. On one occasion she considered becoming a clinical psychologist, but after taking several classes, she worried about the potential emotional toll. On another occasion, she returned to nursing school for four months to become a pediatric nurse practitioner. She truly enjoyed working with children in a public health setting. Layoffs and other opportunities resulted in her working at a local psychiatric facility, where she put to use her psychology courses as she tried her hand at psychiatric nursing, finding it something she enjoyed enough to continue doing for the next decade or so.

Anne describes herself as a very independent person, and she joked that she never wanted anyone to tell her what hours she had to work. A perpetual free spirit, Anne decided to return to the academic setting once more, this time to become a creative writer. She completed her second bachelor's degree, this time in English, and then followed that degree with a master's in humanities. This time, the education was simply for her and for her love of learning. She didn't have a family to whom she was responsible, and her lifestyle allowed her to follow her dreams. She joined a literary club and wrote parts of a novel, all the while supporting herself through her nursing skills. She wrote about what she knew. She was raised in a Polish-American family in a small town, and she wrote parts of her story through the voice of a child. Interwoven throughout the story were her life, her thoughts, and her family. She loves to write, Anne told me, but for some reason, the novel was never finished, and had gotten packed away to gather dust. Anne had retired a few months before I met her. "Someday I'll get back to that," she told me. But for now, it was visiting with Katie that consumed most of her time.

Anne was able to volunteer with Katie at the same hospital where she had worked during her last few years. After working a full day, she would drive to the nearby home where Katie stayed during the day, and together they would return to the hospital to bring smiles to those they visited. Once Anne retired, she continued on as a volunteer with Katie, and especially enjoys working with the physical therapist. One memorable patient was a twelve-year-old girl who had been in physical therapy most of her life due to her cerebral palsy. Eager to make the physical therapy fun, the therapist incorporated Katie into the work, asking the child to unbuckle and buckle her collar and vest, throw the ball, or take Katie for a walk with Anne. By simply adding a therapy dog to the routine, the child became more energized and willing to complete the activities. She was even a guest speaker to other therapy dog teams as she proudly showed the new teams how Katie helps her.

But it was Anne and Katie's work at the children's residential treatment program that touched me the most, for there they meet with two specially selected girls each week. Although they work without a therapist present, Anne is assigned a general goal for their work with each child. For example, one of the first children with whom they worked was a twelve-year-old girl who had difficulty bonding. The hope was that if the child could learn to bond with a therapy dog, this skill could then generalize to other areas of her life. With ten months of weekly visiting ahead, they had plenty of time to forge a relationship, and when the time came to say good-bye, the bond was clearly apparent. The young girl looked sadly into Katie's eyes and then said to Anne, "She looks so sad. She's sad because this is our last visit." Through working with Katie, she had learned it was safe to open her heart once again. It was hard for Anne to say good-bye as well.

It was through working with these children, wanting to make a meaningful difference, that Anne got an idea. She had recently heard Dr. Aubrey Fine speak about the personalized stationery that he had created for use in his own practice with his therapy dogs, and she instantly knew this would make a difference for those she visited as well. She began to design stationery for Katie with rubber stamps and pictures, and soon she was penning letters from Katie to give to the children they visited.

On one occasion, a deeply disturbed child lived in one of the dorms Anne and Katie visited. The child made a high pitched cackling sound and could not communicate in the conventional way. Katie was immediately perplexed, and then she turned for the door. Sensitive to Katie's needs, Anne left the dorm and did not visit at that location until the child was moved to a facility that could better meet her needs. When Anne did return to the dorm to visit with another resident, Susan, Katie instantly remembered and was leery; thinking maybe that scary child was just around the corner. After hearing why Katie was spooked, Susan took it upon herself to comfort Katie and help her relax and feel safe. She then began to gently massage Katie, and soon Katie understood she was safe and enjoyed the visits. After one such visit, Anne wrote the following letter:

Dear Susan,

My mom's been experimenting with making my own stationery so I can write some of my favorite people. She'll continue working on it so my color is a little more true to me. I look a little sick, don't you think [referring to a picture in the right hand corner of the stationery]? But I don't want to hurt her feelings, so I told her I didn't think you'd mind if it's not perfect, especially because I wanted to write the letter to give you on our visit tomorrow.

I want to say thank you for being so gentle with me and helping me to relax. As you know, I had a pretty bad experience in your dorm and got so scared I pulled my mom right out the door. My mom says I might be a little too sensitive, but she knows me well and says she won't put me in a situation I can't handle. I think you understand me pretty well, too.

I like it when you give me a massage (or rub down). I hear you learned to do it with your work with horses. I bet they liked it, too. You have a very special touch and seem to know just the right thing to do.

I hope your visit with your mom went well. Mom says if the weather is nice tomorrow, you'll take me for a walk. I like to pull and sniff along the way, but I'll try not to pull too hard.

Your Pet Partner friend and therapy dog,

Katie

As Anne told me about the letters she had been writing to the children from Katie, there was a twinkle in her eyes that told me how much she enjoyed this. "It's gotten me back to my creative writing," she disclosed, almost by happenstance. As Anne continued to rattle on about various experiences during their visits, my mind began to trail off as I realized what I had just discovered. It was the answer to my question of how Katie had changed Anne. Katie had found a way to integrate Anne's love of creative writing into their special time together. Although it was not through finishing the novel that Anne had ambitiously started years before, it was through a much more special avenue, one that touched young girls' hearts one by one. In writing letters through Katie's voice, Anne is able to send messages of compassion and caring to the children. It is that genuine blending of personal struggles and reflections with the facts of the story that make the letters so irresistible to put down, letters that touch young girls' hearts forever.

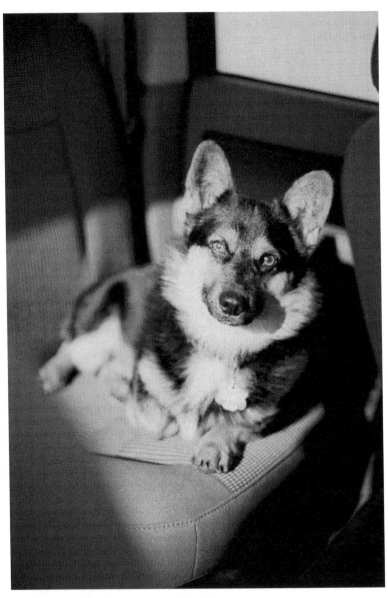

Mr. Big
*Photo by Jodi Geis*

# Chapter Sixteen
# Mr. Big

*There is no psychiatrist in the world
like a puppy licking your face.*

—Bern Williams

Grief. It is an unwelcome emotion that sooner or later visits us all. It may come after a missed opportunity, or after a much larger life tragedy such as the loss of a loved one. We may not know when it will come, but it comes to us all in time. One of the characteristics that makes grief hard to bear is that it often comes disguised as a different emotion such as joy, only to rear its ugly head in time. Such was the story of Jodi.

It was a warm summer day in 2005 when Jodi's stepdaughter ran into the house proudly announcing that she had "saved" a puppy from a boy at school. The boy's family was unable to care for the litter and was trying to find homes for the tiny pups. The puppy was a mixed breed, the sort often referred to as a common mutt. Jodi was used to animals. She had been raised on a ranch and had been around them all her life. When she married, it was to a man who was in the cattle/horse business, and they depended on animals for a living. Animals were always a part of her world. She already had one dog, and its place was outdoors with all of the other animals. So when she saw this helpless creature, she knew she had to do something to help. The puppy was clearly too young to have been weaned. Jodi's stepdaughters took the little pup in and did their best to nurse her back to health. On occasion, Jodi even allowed the puppy (whom she named Harley) into the house when no one was around. Over time, she fell in love with the little dog and developed a relationship with her that she had never experienced with a canine before.

It was then, when Jodi had let her guard down and begun to love this dog, that the painful emotion of grief reared its ugly head. Four or five months after Harley had first arrived, she began to have uncontrollable seizures. And one day Harley died from those seizures in Jodi's arms. Her grief was inconsolable. Her husband, so used to being able to help any animal on his ranch, was helpless to help his wife's little pup. To this day, the clothes that she was wearing that horrible day hang in Jodi's closet with the stains and reminders of those events. Grief is so much harder to bear when it first comes disguised as joy.

Desperate to help her sister through her grief, Jodi's sister, Melanie, insisted that they go to a pet store in a neighboring town to pick out another dog. Jodi was willing to go, but was not in agreement about getting another dog. No one could ever replace little Harley. Accompanied by Jodi's nieces, Reesa and Katelin, the sisters looked at each puppy in the store. All were adorable. What puppy isn't? Then Reesa spotted a cute little corgi schipperke mix. He was black with brown accents, a stubby tail, tiny ears standing straight up, and he weighed only a few pounds. "He's the one!" Reesa cried excitedly. "You have to take him!" she pleaded. It wasn't the dog that Jodi would have picked out. She was partial to chocolate labs, and she couldn't help but notice that there was one there in that very pet store. But unable to resist Reesa's pleas, Jodi left the pet store that day with the little corgi schipperke mix.

Jodi named her new pet Mr. Big; such a big name for such a little pup. He had a big job ahead—to heal Jodi's broken heart. For some reason, Jodi broke her own rules about having dogs in the house. He even slept on her bed at night. With time, Mr. Big slowly chased grief away from Jodi, and began the healing. He became her little buddy.

Jodi began reading training books and even enrolled in an obedience class with Mr. Big. She worked with him between classes, and together they learned the needed lessons to function well in the community as a team. Then one day during a professional conference, Jodi heard about therapy dogs and the incredible work they do. She was intrigued. As a licensed professional counselor for a community mental health center for the past eight years, she knew well the difficulty professionals encounter in engaging and working with the clients who need assistance. She immediately knew that this idea held some promise. After some research, she discovered an organization called Therapy Dogs Incorporated in Wyoming. Soon she was working with a representative from the organization, and she and Mr. Big were being evaluated to ensure that they had the necessary skills and temperament to be registered as a therapy dog team. Mr. Big was a natural, and they passed with flying colors.

After passing the exam, Jodi found herself in the exciting position of proposing to the community mental health center that Mr. Big become a part of their team. Working in a rural setting was an advantage to Jodi's proposal. Limited resources and a more relaxed environment necessitate creativity in rural communities. The community mental health center was already known for its innovation, having already approved horticulture and art therapy groups. Adding a canine to the treatment mix only seemed to make sense, since animals were so central to the lives of their clientele.

Mr. Big was an instant hit with both the clients and the staff members. Mr. Big clearly enjoyed his work, and he greeted each person he visited with enthusiasm as he wagged his stubby tail. As Jodi stated, "He just brings joy." Having Mr. Big as a co-worker opened countless doors for Jodi with her clients. Many of her clients have had a life of hardship and pain. Many of them have never experienced joy. On one occasion, Jodi took her clients and their children to the local park to "teach them what joy feels like." What better teacher than Mr. Big? With minimal effort, he soon had each client smiling and laughing at his antics. Jodi quickly learned that sitting on the floor (the best position for clients and staff to easily interact with Mr. Big due to his tiny size) had an amazing effect on the therapy sessions. The dynamics instantly changed, interactions were more spontaneous, and formality was greatly reduced. All of which had a surprising positive impact on the therapy results. Often the unassuming addition of physical contact with another living creature seemed to calm the clients and ground them in reality. Jodi discovered that the simple act of having Mr. Big sit on a developmentally delayed client's lap and allowing him to lick the woman's face could open doors that she, with all her professional credentials, could not otherwise open.

During one visit, Jodi was working with a child who was fearful of getting a physical exam from a doctor. Jodi instantly had an idea. Before long Jodi and the child were practicing the physical exam on Mr. Big, checking his blood pressure with a pressure cuff, checking his reflexes, and more, all to the delight of the young child. Mr. Big was just happy to be a part of the game. He happily wagged his stubby tail to encourage the smiles and laughter. Due to Jodi and Mr. Big's efforts, the child's physical exam was completed with minimal concern on the part of the child and to the relief of the adults. Mr. Big has an uncanny way of helping Jodi address a myriad of issues including self-esteem, trust, and handling emotions.

"Pets are a commonality," Jodi explains. Animals are one thing many of us have in common, and they bond us together. Having a therapy dog in the office grants Jodi instant rapport with many clients and lends some clients to think, "You're cool. You're a dog lover." Over the course of time Jodi has attracted several dog sitters (co-workers who love to have Mr. Big visit in their offices when Jodi needs to work with a client without him), and some even have jokingly expressed hurt feelings when they aren't chosen to watch Mr. Big when needed. While she has found it helpful to initially meet with clients without Mr. Big in order to screen for the appropriateness of therapy dog intervention (not everyone is a dog person), she frequently includes him in her sessions when it is clinically appropriate. Now other therapists even ask her to bring the dog to occasional sessions with their clients. Jodi tells me that the employees are happier now that Mr. Big has joined the team, and many ask her, "Where's Mr. Big today?" when he has a day off.

Mr. Big had such a significant impact on Jodi that she returned to the pet store to learn more about his history. It was then that she learned that he was the runt of the litter of a Kansas breeder that had sold him to the puppy broker. After Jodi located this breeder, she purchased a second puppy, who she named Isabella Big ("so that she could be called Mrs. Big," she explained with a smile). She has high hopes for Isabella (Izzy for short), but acknowledges that she will need some training before she is ready to follow in Mr. Big's paw prints. The two pups are the best of friends, and they clearly have Jodi wrapped around their paws—she beamed with pride as I visited with them both. To see her with her two little pups, I never would have guessed that she was ever a person who believed that a dog's place was outdoors. Mr. and Mrs. Big have changed her thinking on that, for sure!

In addition to adding Izzy to the family, Jodi decided to breed Mr. Big with a co-worker's corgi. Two months later, Mr. Big was the proud papa to four adorable puppies. As part of the breeding agreement, Jodi was given the pick of the litter, which she in turn gave to an office mate at the community mental health center. It is their dream that someday Mr. Big's daughter will grow up to be a therapy dog at the center, just like her dad.

It is a life that Jodi never had considered—breeding and working with therapy dogs. However, it is a life that has truly changed her to her core. During my talk with Jodi and her niece, Reesa, they laughed as they told me how different Jodi is today because of Mr. Big. Before Mr. Big, Jodi was a self-proclaimed "neat freak." Everything needed to be tidied up and in its place. Mr. and Mrs. Big have changed all that! She is now less preoccupied with the little things in day-to-day life, and is more comfortable with the tufts of wafting dog fur, normal stains, and dirty paws that are an everyday occurrence when one loves a dog. Mr. and Mrs. Big have taught her about the power of the human-animal bond and shown her that animals can truly touch one's heart. She now loves animals on a level that was previously unimaginable, and is more sensitive to those around her. As I listened to her talk, I could not help but envision a more spontaneous and relaxed way of life as she told me that she now enjoys traveling with her little canines, and has discovered the joy of pet-friendly motels (something that she previously didn't even know existed). "What a wonderful way to meet people you wouldn't otherwise meet!" she explained.

As we chatted about the difference she has noticed since Mr. Big came into her life, she told me what a difficult period she was going through when Harley died. In addition to the loss of her little friend, she was unhappy in her job as a supervisor at the mental health center. She missed clinical work, and was discovering that management did not give her joy. It was an important, but painful, lesson. Mr. Big played an important role in not only healing her grief, but also in providing the pathway back into meaningful clinical work once she returned to a position as a frontline therapist.

Now, when grief and other painful emotions come near, Mr. and Mrs. Big bring her joy. They distract her from the tediousness of life, and give her comfort and laughter. They keep her from getting lonely when her husband travels and keep her house feeling like a home full of love. While grief is an emotion that will inevitably visit us all from time to time, Jodi has now found a way to heal from its wounds. It is a way that she happily shares with her clients in hope that joy will someday replace the grief in their hearts as it has in her own.

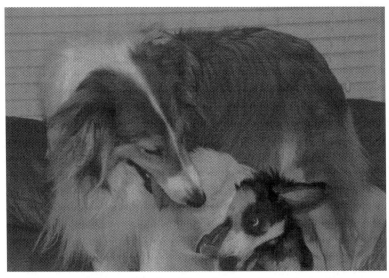

Rocky and Jasper Playing Shortly after We Adopted Jasper
*Photo by Mark Hochstedler*

# Epilogue
# The Gift of the Imperfect Dog

*It's funny how dogs and cats*
*know the inside of folks better*
*than other folks do.*

—Eleanor H. Potter

My dogs have a way of humbling me. As part of my "day job" I frequently take one of my boys to the administrative building and speak to new employees during orientation about the work we do. Seasoned employees are also required to attend every few years as a way to keep them informed about changes that may have occurred without their knowledge. Only twenty or so employees attend these presentations, and the room is relatively small. I typically close the door and allow the therapy dog to informally greet audience members as I talk, once I am assured that everyone would enjoy an up-close greeting. I normally take Rocky on such excursions since he has a reputation as a charmer, and has an uncanny gift of working the crowd. He somehow knows who he has visited and who has not yet been graced by his presence, skillfully backtracking to ensure all have ample opportunity to gaze into his beautiful eyes and stroke his soft fur. However, on this particular day, I decided to bring Jasper instead in an effort to expose him to different settings and tasks.

Jasper did an excellent job meeting and greeting employees on our way through the office corridors, and eagerly demonstrated his skill by balancing a bone on his nose before effortlessly catching it and savoring each crumb, all to the delight of on-lookers. Once in the conference room, I began my presentation; educating attendees about the values of animal-assisted activities/ therapy, all the while stressing the amount of time and effort the therapy dogs require in order to ensure that dogs and people are safe and the dogs remain well behaved. It was then—right when I was speaking about his impeccable manners and solid obedience skills—that I spied Jasper with his front paws on the shoulders of his dear friend, Donna, who was crouched on the floor enjoying doggie kisses on her checks and ear lobes. Unfortunately, this was one of those occasions during which my words continued to tumble out of my mouth despite my sudden realization that Jasper was well-intentionally violating several therapy dog rules in his effort to ensure that Donna received all the snuggle time she desired. Needless to say, I was unable to stop mid-sentence. I directed everyone's attention toward Jasper's obedience/qualification patches, carefully sewn onto his vest. The only problem was that the dog who was at that moment wearing the vest was not living up to what the patches represented. This was clearly not one of those Kodak moments from the front of a therapy dog brochure. Although both Donna and Jasper were thoroughly enjoying each other's company, this was not the example of appropriate therapy dog behavior that I was looking for. As the room erupted into laughter and I gently reminded my canine partner to keep all four paws on the ground unless performing a requested trick, I was reminded that it is often the "human" side of our dogs that truly endear them to those they visit.

When I was a child, I had a wonderful toy poodle named J.J. (her actual name was Poodle Town's Black Jade Princess, but that was far too complex for a two-year-old, so J.J. it was). She was an outdoor dog, and I spent countless hours in our California backyard enjoying each minute with her. I really can't remember any problems we ever had with J.J. She was the perfect dog for a child; she allowed me to dress her up in doll clothes and push her down the street in my doll carriage. I used to marvel how this little dog could be so perfect when we never once took her to an obedience class or took the time to socialize her appropriately. I now realize that, while I truly enjoyed my little friend, her perfection led me to take her for granted in many ways.

Lassie (Knight, 1938) was my favorite childhood hero, most likely paving the way for a lifelong love of rough coat collies. I dreamed of having such a regal and perfect dog as a companion. This desire to have the perfect dog continued as I watched therapy dogs flawlessly perfect each task, ignoring temptations with apparent ease. I heard countless stories about dogs who were perfect from the start and took to therapy work as though it was what they had been born to do. So many handlers described an effortless process on their path to working in partnership together. When I got Rocky and then later Jasper, I was initially disappointed to discover that my canine friends did not have this natural ability from the start. My quest for the perfect dog eluded me. I then decided that my destiny lay on the path of hard work, so I began the journey to patiently and tirelessly help them past their imperfections toward the path of success. It was somewhere down this difficult and challenging road that I began to realize the real work that needed to be done was in me.

One of my favorite parts of my day job is teaching inexperienced therapists how to truly hear and respect clients and, ultimately, how to skillfully ask purposeful questions that invite and guide lasting change. It is commonplace for these new therapists to slowly build self-confidence, only to later become disillusioned when they encounter a client with whom their skills seemed to utterly fail. While the therapists' initial response is frequently to blame some aspect of the client ("He doesn't want to change," "He's inappropriate for treatment," and the like), it is at this point in their professional development that they have the greatest opportunity for growth. At such times, I explain that there are two general classifications of clients: easy clients (those who are very forgiving of therapist's blunders and lack of purpose and make changes despite these factors) and difficult clients (those who unwittingly expose every therapist mistake and therapeutic guess and force the therapists to sharpen their skills and be more purposeful and precise). I often tell therapists that I am glad when they are working with one of these "difficult clients," for it is those who truly challenge one's skills that force us to choose— blame the client or to hone our skills.

In working with my two imperfect dogs, I am forced to be much more aware than I would otherwise have to be. Rocky is painfully tuned into my moods, so he quickly shows discomfort when I become frustrated and impatient. He is a barometer of my mood and an ever-present reminder of personal aspects that I would be wise to improve. Jasper is incredibly mindful of my body position, and instinctively takes his cues from how I move rather than from what I say. In doing so, he forces me to take responsibility for those moments when I am not congruent. In addition, the dogs' quirks and oddities force me to carefully screen the environment and be mindful of their interpretations and signals. They are in many ways high maintenance. While these things used to frustrate me, I have come to value the lessons they have brought to my life. I now realize that because of my partners' quirks I have become a far better handler and human being than I most likely would have been had I been working with less sensitive and more easy-going canine partners.

As I reflect upon my favorite childhood dog, I realize that, while the story of Lassie was heartwarming and entertaining, this was not a book in which Timmy walked away with any lasting revelations or personal self-improvement. A perfect dog does not inspire such self-reflection. On the other hand, stories about dogs with issues or behavioral problems, such as Jon Katz's (2003, 2006) Orson or John Grogan's (2005) Marley, are not only entertaining but are riddled with self-reflections and realizations that can only conclude with a wiser human being, leaving both human and dog better because of the other. For it is in being in relationship with such an imperfect dog that one has to choose—blame or even get rid of the dog (or one's dreams), or to learn to be a better human being. This is the gift of the imperfect dog. It is my wish that someday you will be blessed with such an imperfect dog.

# Appendix A
Suggested Reading

Aloff, B. (2005). *Canine body language: A photographic guide.* Wenatchee, WA: Dogwise.

Beck, A., & Katcher, A. (1996). *Between pets and people.* West Lafayette, IN: Purdue University.

Burch, M. R. (1996). *Volunteering with your pet: How to get involved in animal-assisted therapy with any kind of pet.* New York: Howell Book House.

Clothier, S. (2002). *Bones would rain from the sky: Deepening our relationships with dogs.* New York: Warner.

Coren, S. (2000). *How to speak dog: Mastering the art of dog-human communication.* New York: Fireside.

Crawford, J. J., & Pomerinke, K. A. (2003). *Therapy pets: The animal-human healing partnership.* Amherst, NY: Prometheus.

Cusack, O., & Smith, E. (Eds.). (1984). *Pets and the elderly: The therapeutic bond.* New York: Haworth.

Davis, K. D. (2002). *Therapy dogs: Training your dog to reach others* (2nd ed.). Wenatchee, WA: Dogwise.

Delta Society (May 2003). *Animal-assisted therapy (AAT) applications I student guide.* (No. AAT-711). Renton, WA: Author.

Delta Society. (1997). *Therapeutic interventions* (No. AAT253). Renton, WA: Author.

Delta Society. (1996). *Standards of practice* (No. AAT251). Renton, WA: Author.

Dibra, B. (1999). *Dog speak: How to learn it, speak it, and use it to have a happy, healthy, well-behaved dog.* New York: Fireside.

Donaldson, J. (1996). *The culture clash.* Oakland: James & Kenneth Publishers.

Dunbar, I. (1991). *How to teach a new dog old tricks.* Oakland: Kenneth & James.

Dunbar, I. (1979). *Dog behavior.* Neptune, NJ: T.H.F. Publications, Inc.

Fine, A. H. (2006). *Animal-assisted therapy: Theoretical Foundations and guidelines for practice.* San Diego: Academic Press.

Fine, A. H. & C. J. Eisen. (2008). *Afternoons with puppy: Inspirations from a therapist and his animals.* West Lafayette, IN: Purdue University.

Friedmann, E., Katcher, A. H., Lynch, J. J., & Thomas, S. A. (1980). "Animal companions and one-year survival of patients after discharge from a coronary care unit." *Public Health Reports, 95,* 307-12.

Friedmann, E., Katcher, A. H., Thomas, S. A., Lynch, J. J., & Messent, P. R. (1983). "Social interaction and blood pressure." *Journal of Nervous and Mental Disease, 171,* 461-465.

Gerben, R. (2003). "Kids + dogs = combination for paw-rrific reading adventures." *Interactions, 21*(2), 4-8.

Haggerty, C. (2000). *How to teach your dog to talk.* New York: Fireside.

Howie, A. R. (Ed.). (2000). *The pet partners team training course* (5th ed.). Renton, WA: Delta Society.

Intermountain Therapy Animals (2003-2004). *Reading education assistance dogs training manual.* Salt Lake City, UT: Author.

Katz, J. (2007). *Dog days.* New York: Villard.

Katz, J. (2006). *A good dog.* New York: Villard.

Katz, J. (2005). *Katz on dogs.* New York: Villard.

Katz, J. (2004). *The dogs of bedlam farm.* New York: Villard.

Katz, J. (2003). *A dog year: Twelve months, four dogs, and me.* New York: Random House.

Katz, J. (2003). *The new work of dogs.* New York: Villard.

McNicholas, J., & Collis, G. M. (1995). "The end of a relationship: Coping with pet loss." In I. Robinson (Ed.), *The Waltham book of human-animal interaction: Benefits and responsibilities of pet-ownership* (pp. 127-143). Oxford: Pergamon.

The Monks of New Skete. (2003). *I & dog.* New York: Yorkville Press.

The Monks of New Skete. (2002). *How to be your dog's best friend* (2nd ed.). New York: Little Brown.

Pichot, T. & Coulter, M. (2007). *Animal-assisted brief therapy: A solution-focused approach.* New York: Taylor & Francis.

Pryor, K. (1999). *Don't shoot the dog (revised).* North Bend: Sunshine Books.

Rugaas, T. (1997). *On talking terms with dogs: Calming signals.* Sequim, WA: Legacy Publications.

Serpell, J. A. (1996). *In the company of animals* (2nd ed.) Cambridge: Cambridge University Press.

Siegel, J. M. (1980). "Stressful life events and use of physician services among the elderly: The moderating role of pet ownership." *Journal of Personality and Social Psychology,* 58, 1081-1086.

Sussman M. B. (Ed.). (1985). *Pets and the family.* New York: Haworth.

Tillman, P. (2000). *Clicking with your dog.* Waltham, MA: Sunshine Books.

Wilkes, G. (1995). *The click and treat starter kit* (with video). North Blend: Sunshine Books.

Wilson, C. C., & Turner, D. C. (Eds.). (1998). *Companion animals in human health.* Thousand Oaks, CA: Sage.

# Appendix B
National/International Therapy Dog Organizations


Delta Society
875 – 124th Ave NE, Suite 101
Bellevue, WA 98005-2531
(425) 226-7357
(425) 235-1076 (fax)
info@deltasociety.org
www.deltasociety.org

This organization provides information on the requirements for membership as well as credentialing. Delta provides instructors and training materials to teach the skills needed to visit safely with an animal in hospitals, nursing homes, classrooms, and other facilities. Regular publications keep participants up to date on emerging issues, research, and a wide variety of information on the human-animal bond. With successful completion of the registration requirements, you receive liability insurance, referrals to facilities, newsletters, and continuing education opportunities as well as networking support.

Intermountain Therapy Animals (ITA)
1555 East Statford Avenue
Suite 400
Salt Lake City, UT 84106
(801) 272-3439
www.therapyanimals.org

This organization provides information about how to become credentialed to participate in the Reading Education Assistance Dog (R.E.A.D.) program as well as other information. The mission of the R.E.A.D. program is to improve the literacy skills of children through the assistance of registered Pet Partner therapy teams as literacy mentors.

Therapy Dogs, Inc.
PO Box 5868
Cheyenne, WY 82003
(877) 843-7364
(307) 638-2079 (fax)
therdog@sisna.com
www.therapydogs.com

A goal of Therapy Dogs Inc. is to help dog owners use their dogs for therapy work in various places such as nursing homes, hospitals, and schools, as well as in work with the mentally and physically handicapped.

Therapy Dogs International, Inc.
88 Bartley Road
Flanders, NJ 07836
(973) 252-9800
(973) 252-7171 (fax)
tdi@gti.net
www.tdi-dog.org

Therapy Dogs International, Inc. (TDI) is a volunteer group organized to provide qualified handlers and their therapy dogs for visitations to institutions, facilities, and any other place where therapy dogs are needed.

The St. John's Ambulance Therapy Dogs (Canada)
St. John Ambulance Halton Hills
PO Box 145, Norval
Ontario, Canada

LOP 1K0
(905) 873-8442
(905) 873-7646 fax
www.sja.ca

# Bibliography

Brown, A., & Finkelhor, D. (1986 January). "Impact of child sexual abuse: A review of the research." *Psychological Bulletin, 99*(1):66-77.

Cloud, W., & Granfield (2001). *Recovery from addiction.* New York: New York University Press.

de Shazer, S. (1985). *Keys to solution in brief therapy.* New York: Norton.

de Shazer, S. (1988). *Clues: Investigating solutions in brief therapy.* New York: Norton.

Grogan, J. (2005). *Marley & me: Life and love with the world's worst dog.* New York: Harper.

Katz, J. (2006). *A good dog.* New York: Villard.

Katz, J. (2003). *A dog year: Twelve months, four dogs, and me.* New York: Random House.

Kendler, K. S., Bulik, C. M., Silberg, J., Hettema, J. M., Myers, J., & Prescott, C. A. (2000, October). "Childhood sexual abuse and adult psychiatric and substance use disorders in women." *Archives of General Psychiatry 57*(10):953-959.

Knight, E. (1938). *Lassie come-home.* New York: Holt, Rinehart, and Winston.

Luthar, S. S., Cicchetti, D., & Becker, B. (2000). "The construct of resilience: A critical evaluation and guidelines for future work." *Child Development, 71(3),* 543-562.

Luthar, S. S. & Cicchetti, D. (2000). "The construct of resilience: Implications for interventions and social policies." *Development and Psychopathology, 12,* 857-885.

Schreiber, F. R. R. (1989). Sybil. New York: Grand Central Publishing.